The Performance Therapist and Authentic Therapeutic Identity

I0025036

Exploring what it means to be an authentic therapist in the present day, Sara London playfully melds together the tenets of performance art and psychoanalytic theory to advance the hopeful new notion of the *performance therapist*.

In an era where the therapist is now more of a public-facing entity than ever before, developing a sense of who one is both inside and outside of the consulting room is a complex undertaking. In response, London reconceptualises the therapist's identity in a contemporary way, transcending preconceived labels, by bringing an understanding of performance art into an analysis of psychotherapeutic practice. Through this interdisciplinary approach, London attends to the complex questions faced by psychoanalysts and psychotherapists in training and in practice: can a therapist perform *and* be authentic? Can a therapist perform and have true intimate relationships within the confines of that performance? And can a therapist perform as themselves?

This provocative and highly original work will provide both new and experienced psychotherapists with an understanding of the clinical and philosophical significance of performance art to cultivating therapeutic identity.

Sara London, M.A. is a freelance journalist, author, and satirist-when-convenient. She has a graduate degree in a specialised psychoanalytic research program from New York University's Gallatin School. Additionally, she writes articles about psychology, wellness, pop culture, and the future of work primarily to fund her many hare-brained schemes.

The Performance Therapist and Authentic Therapeutic Identity

Coming into Being

Sara London

Routledge
Taylor & Francis Group

LONDON AND NEW YORK

Designed cover image: Roi and Roi © Getty Images

First published 2024
by Routledge
4 Park Square, Milton Park, Abingdon, Oxon OX14 4RN

and by Routledge
605 Third Avenue, New York, NY 10158

Routledge is an imprint of the Taylor & Francis Group, an informa business

© 2024 Sara London

The right of Sara London to be identified as author of this work has been asserted in accordance with sections 77 and 78 of the Copyright, Designs and Patents Act 1988.

All rights reserved. No part of this book may be reprinted or reproduced or utilised in any form or by any electronic, mechanical, or other means, now known or hereafter invented, including photocopying and recording, or in any information storage or retrieval system, without permission in writing from the publishers.

Trademark notice: Product or corporate names may be trademarks or registered trademarks, and are used only for identification and explanation without intent to infringe.

British Library Cataloguing-in-Publication Data
A catalogue record for this book is available from the British Library

ISBN: 978-1-032-53580-7 (hbk)
ISBN: 978-1-032-53582-1 (pbk)
ISBN: 978-1-003-41269-4 (ebk)

DOI: 10.4324/9781003412694

Typeset in Galliard
by MPS Limited, Dehradun

To Zach and Jess, who, in a way, made this possible.

Contents

Foreword

In order to thoroughly flesh out the meaning and purpose of this work, I've been told I should find my place in it. This is, I've found, quite a bit harder than it seems. Regretfully I deny any deep attachment to categories like "artist" or "Li'l Future Psychoanalyst," or "person who appreciates most of the current installations at the Whitney," as that would make things so easy. I am not an analyst, and I have no analytic training. I am not a therapist, and I have never seen a patient. Oh, but don't stop reading now! I'm a very well-trained analysand, from a long line of Sabina Spielreins and Lou Salomés and other dark-haired women in furs who started their journey laying on the couch, not behind it. A writer who doesn't take myself too seriously, I have written many a piece for many a client, bylines littered about online like breadcrumbs leading back to the trail of my career, trying to bring an element of psychological mindedness to topics like the future of work, business news, and pop culture. Like many others, psychoanalysis has been a lifelong lifestyle for me, and while reading Freud and Kierkegaard made me no friends at the high-school lunch table, it set me up with a foundation of knowledge for my Master's degree in "an intensive psychoanalytic study," as I colloquially call it. But is that my place in the field, to lie on the couch, a book in my arms and a pen in my hand, swooning with hysteria as onlookers toss pennies into my cage until I freely associate some brilliant pearls of wisdom? Sure – it's nice work if you can get it!

Unfortunately for me, I've found that coming from a specific place of expertise tied linearly to a line of work aids in one's arguments about certain things. For instance, the declaration that some foolish amateur improperly dry-brushed their painting of the grassy knoll holds more water if your own fresco of an alien as the second shooter is hanging in the MoMA. This leaves the thinker in an unfortunate position; not the doer, of course, as we thinkers are known mostly to stick to thinking. I've decided that all the thinking I do has rendered me with some good ideas. I suppose that remains to be seen, as I haven't stated a single one yet.

I'll just say this: I come to you seeing what I see, from where I've seen it – from the couch, from behind a book, from my discussions and discourses with many brilliant analysts, psychologists, social workers, and mental health professionals quoted and unquoted, named and anonymous. From my observations of group supervisions and didactics, from lectures, from articles, from social media, from un-social media. Should this work be an incredible success, the credit partially goes to my beloved fiancé, a brilliant clinical psychologist and supervisor, and my beloved analyst, who taught me more about the analytic process than books ever did. I'd also like to express my appreciation for the two young men I met on an Amtrak to Burlington, VT last November – we had four and a half hours to waste chatting on a broken train, and they were quite the conversationalists. Should it be a failure, perhaps it's only because I have four people to thank, and I only really know two of them. I shall blame them all at any rate.

We might seem like we're getting somewhere, but I'm still a bit skeptical.

I understand your hesitancy, believe me. There's a sort of definitiveness about the idea of making claims that does not seem right to me – "I'm a philosopher!" – "I'm a social scientist!" – I am a studier, a looker-at of things, one who swoops in, identifies The Issues, and leaves in a hurry, throwing my smoke bomb, whipping my cape around and disappearing into the night. I always thought there was something tired about that, and the exhausting cliché that everyone's a critic has become an exhausting reality. One who wishes to say something they find important and meaningful has their message washed away by the deluge of discourse and finds themselves making a commentary about commentary in the forward of their own commentary. Oh, the humanity!

But what do I seek to do, to accomplish? I started with a graduate thesis, the trajectory of which has changed exponentially since my first draft, as these things tend to go. I spent three years in that program poring over content and immersing myself in the therapeutic world, and an additional two years after graduation turning that exploration into a more fleshed-out manifesto. But that puts me in a rather funky spot. I am neither in the ivory tower with a Professor Emeritus tramp stamp, hurling barbs of condescension at the less educated, nor am I the grime-covered, degreeless chump, wearing only a barrel, yelling from the gutter as professionals scoff at my ramblings with alacrity. Hopefully, I know neither everything nor nothing and acknowledge the grey area of inquisition without denunciation. The ultimate "view from without" – without even having a license, a place in the dialogue, or for that matter, a straightforward forward on why I'm doing it! And *there's* the niche, there's where we begin to understand my urgent necessity to write such a thing. To admit that I know nothing, not even myself, but that I wish to attempt to know – or something like that – and that I wish to bring others into the fold with me. Surely a professional writer could eloquently phrase a consuming, near-radical idea about exploring the mind compounded with the insurmountable urge to share it. I, myself, cannot. At least not at the moment.

I'll give you your answer, the honest answer about why I'm writing this manifesto. I would hope that one wants to understand themselves, and their role not just as a therapist, but a mindful therapist, an integrated therapist, a *performance therapist*, in the same way I would want to understand what I'm all about. "Know thyself," and all that hooey. Or begin to conceptualize what it means to know thyself. Or begin to believe you'll one day conceptualize what it means to know thyself. The process of writing this manifesto has been an informative and difficult one, especially because the content is so deeply personal – a discussion of identity, of authenticity, of performance and of being. In many ways, this book is my "*Two Analyses of Mr. Z*" – I'm a scholar and a patient, an analysand and a researcher, a neurotic and an academic (though those usually aren't too different). I examine every claim as I would in session, wondering with the utmost curiosity if I'm witnessing a projection or an insight. Sometimes the answer is both. And I believe that without an internal compass pointing a therapist towards their own individualized therapeutic identity, their practice and patients very well may suffer. I'm not looking to point one's internal compass in one direction or another, but to aid in its discovery in the first place.

Unfortunately, I believe I've answered nothing, and maybe even muddled the issue even further. Perhaps that's how we should begin.

Introduction

In the words of Tristan Tzara's Dadaist Manifesto, "I write a manifesto and I want nothing, yet to say certain things. And in principle I am against manifestoes, as I am also against principles."

In an era where the therapist's identity is now more of a public-facing entity than it ever was before, developing a sense of who they are both inside and outside the frame is a complex undertaking. Some act out in stark, self-disclosing contrast to the silent, medicalized American analysts of the 1940s,[1] some loyal traditionalists cringe at the idea of having any online presence, and some young therapists aren't sure who they are in the first place. With such disparate theories about the "correct" way to conceptualize one's professional identity, a new discussion must take place regarding who this brave new therapist is as they face the brave new world we find ourselves in. And though this assertion may be dogmatic, it's safe to say that without posing the question of identity – without at least beginning to investigate how we see the therapist both in theory and in our own psychic realms – therapists establish themselves as hypocrites, shutting off exactly what they expect patients, clients, and analysands to be endlessly open to: a discussion of who someone is and why they are that way.

Prior discourses on the therapist's identity usually begin with a more matter-of-fact, sometimes chronological account of one's training, experience, successes, and failures. Ah yes, identity! An amalgamation of what you know, how you know it, and how you express it. In psychoanalytic circles, students also have a particular collective experience around choosing the right analytic school, the right postdoctoral program, the right supervisor, the right buddies in the right cohort. But there seems to be a lack of exploration into what exactly is at stake in discussing the identity of a therapist outside of those definitions, and more creative endeavors that explore the philosophical nature of the field with emotional and verbal nuance often turn into esoteric gobbledygook fit to be decoded only by the sharpest minds. While a therapist may practice for years with a broad and stable sense of identity, clear on how to monitor their countertransference and act well-trained yet reflective with the patient, it can be difficult to put into words. Here, we have the opportunity

DOI: 10.4324/9781003412694-1

for an extended written look into the many different processes behind the therapist's development – a slow-motion peek into the evolution of one's practice. It's one thing to say, "therapeutic identity is complicated, and let's explore it." It's another to say, "the therapist is like a performance artist in their behaviors, thoughts, and processes – and let's explore it."

Ah, but I've buried the lead, haven't I! Performance art and identity, though I'm sure that was relatively evident from the title of the book. Bear with me and we'll get there together.

Those who believe psychology is a science have, at this point, thrown the book across the room at the sheer mention of art. Art, in *my* psychology? *Obscene!* And so, the bickering begins, like two children fighting over a toy. The therapist is an artist, one side usually says, as there is no one so capable of relaying such a deep, intense mélange of practices, ideas, and connections as the artist. There is no way to turn intricate transferential relationships into methodologies, to state goals and measurable outcomes of enactments, to capture the therapeutic alliance in a z-score. But he must be a scientist, the other side retorts! As no one could possibly intellectualize the human mind without the fundamental tenets of science: hypotheses, curiosity, distance and boundaries, exploration, and discovery. Art is not measurable; art is a matter of speculation. And if therapy becomes a matter of speculation, there's no hope for positive outcomes, as every case can be constantly debated until the end of time.

But let's not get too hasty – science-lovers, fear not, as there is hope for your side yet. The therapist is like a performance artist in their behaviors, thoughts, and processes – *performance* being the key word, not artist. When we get down to brass tacks, therapeutic work is not strictly artistic, nor is it strictly scientific, as life is a gray area, nuance is everywhere, etcetera, etcetera (as we all know all too well). Ultimately, a psychoanalytic mind finds comfort in processing ambiguity, and we must apply that notion not only to the inside of the therapy room, but in our own literature and discussion. What a therapist does is something partially informed by an artistic milieu, but not exclusive to the artistic world – they are the canvas and their patient's brush strokes stick to them, creating a slightly different painting with every session. And like a scientist, they take in data, measure it and go over it in their own minds, throwing hypotheses about the roots of trauma or neurosis to the wall, seeing if any stick. The therapist is a student of everything and nothing, the student of art and science, the artist who both is and isn't even an artist. And when the tables are set and the office door is open, the patient brings in their ingredients to co-create the greatest meal they'll ever eat with the chef of the century: **the performance therapist**. But how, then, can the therapist's identity be conceptualized as a performance artist? And who is, then, this mysterious performance therapist?

Before we take off our pool noodles and start swimming laps in the Olympic pool of personhood, we should have some idea of how we're going about this odd exploration. Discerning the identity of the "performance therapist" is but one solution to a more pressing question: *what is the identity of the therapist in 2022?* This comparison is perfect for the modern therapist because the world we live in is hardly one of veritable, constant truth. Performance is everywhere – from conversations over coffee to boardrooms and Zoom calls to the very computer I write this manifesto on. And performance art creates a broader definition of performance in general – it's not just about acting or "being real and fake," it's about turning beliefs into expression. It blurs the line between performance and authenticity and exists in the middle of "real and fake;" yes, right next to the therapist, who knows ambiguity better than anyone.

If performance art is about expressing beliefs, then psychoanalysis is how we can think about understanding what those beliefs mean to us; in a way, psychoanalysis explains who we are, and performance art explains how we show it to the world. And by knowing performance (through, of course, the tenants of performance art), by knowing how a therapist acts, acts out, enacts, wants to be seen, and attempts to be perceived, they thereby know themselves. And by knowing oneself, the very authentic drives, wishes, and fears within your psyche, then things about your therapeutic practice begin coming to light. You can see when you act prohibitively to a patient, thereby impeding their ability to speak freely. You can see when your performance of confidence falls flat, and your ability to hold the frame wavers. You can see moments of countertransference before they hit a volatile intensity. And you become the best version of yourself as a therapist. Perhaps these claims are all heretofore unsubstantiated. But by the end of this work, we'll substantiate them all.

Now, back to this old thing you're reading. We've come to the more practical matter of how we'll be connecting two disparate ideas to form one cohesive identity. If you're sold on the concept of this little fête, we should probably discuss the menu. Appetizers – Part I: Performance Art – are served in the garden of conjecture. Next, we'll have Part II: Identity in the intrapsychic realm, Part III: Performance (or secondi, a bit of pasta) in the therapy room, Part IV: Authenticity in the external world, and finally, a tasty dessert of Part V: Application in the garden of conjecture once more.

In a bit more detail, the layout is as such: first, the history of performance art is explored in a bit of a straightforward crash-course. It's imperative to at least have a semi-solid background in the concept and development of the medium over the ages, and a loose sense of its sociocultural status currently for a number of reasons. While performance art is merely a tool we use to look at the therapist, we need it to become immersed in the world of the therapist's identity. It paints the picture of the psychological fantasyland we're about to enter – one of high drama and high camp, one of deep feelings and exuberant expressions, one of passions and pain, much like the intrapsychic landscape.

Once we have somewhat of a firm foundation of knowledge to build from, we can begin to look at the *performance* part of performance art in and of itself as a psychoanalytic thing. To most, performance is simply the act of getting on a stage, reciting lines, and playing a character. But there's more to performance than just how (or rather, if) someone acts. And to prevent us from remaining mired in our preconceived notions about performance, we shall begin to think of performance as a feature of identity or the "self" by looking at what performance is and how it differs or overlaps with identity. With our pasta, we're going to attempt to define performance in a psychoanalytic way including how one performs psychologically and emotionally. Can one perform in ways that are and aren't like who they see themselves to be? While one can utilize really any psychological theory to do this kind of investigation into the roots of selfhood, this work is a psychoanalytic one, meaning that we'll be learning what it means to perform and be authentic by way of Jung, Winnicott, and Horney.

After our little jaunt into identity, we're all through with foundational knowledge, and we move onto the more experimental part of our work: Part III. Knowing what we will about the nature of performance art and the psychoanalytic framework of identity, we'll be able to break down a therapeutic practice into its bare essentials and fundamental components. Rather than talking about a performance artist, we'll start talking about a performance therapist, one who both performs as a therapist and *is* a therapist. What are the building blocks of their performance? The integral parts of their therapeutic identity's scope? And once we discover the components of a performance therapist as they stand alone, what about when we bring the patient into the picture? How does one's therapeutic identity warp and change when confronted with the identity of another?

In Part VI, the elephant in the room is introduced with much enthusiasm – we've talked for pages about performance, but only skimmed over authenticity, its' supposed antithesis. We're not quite sure what it is, but we give the definition a go regardless. And then, we extrapolate this definition to the therapist, from their perspective alone. What does is a 'real relationship' from the therapist's perspective, and does it indicate a certain level of authenticity? Does self-disclosure constitute authenticity in one's therapeutic identity? Authenticity is then taken out of its' vacuum, alone in the therapist's mind, and pontificated upon within the working alliance. And what about when the therapist steps out of the session, yet must maintain the performance of the mental health professional – what then?

And finally, we find ourselves back in the garden of conjecture, figuring out how to apply it all in Part V. This performance-art-alytic stew, with its intoxicating aromas and subtle flavors, simmer into new notes of theoretical importance. We must have ourselves a little tasting to delineate what exactly this identity means, and to pick apart all sides of it, including what it is not. Can a therapist perform *and* be authentic? Can they perform and have true intimate relationships within the confines of that performance? And can one perform as themselves?

Finally, we'll conclude with a sort of abbreviated symposium on the philosophical implications of making such a claim – of redefining, or of attempting to redefine something that can be so ambiguous. A performance therapist's masterwork, if executed with intentionality, results in the intimately beautiful experience of the therapeutic relationship, the magic of relating, or what we call a "coming into being" (the title, if you've forgotten). Our meal will have resulted in a depiction of balancing performance and authenticity leading to a strong sense of professional identity. And a way to understand the modern therapist will be revealed.

Then we all split the bill and go home. But do come back any time – though the *carte du jour* is more of a *carte tous les jours*, you always know what you'll be getting.

The guest list

Despite the fact that we'll be talking mostly about psychoanalysis (evidenced by the fact that most of the literature cited in this book refers to analysts and analytic cases), this work is actually *not* just for the trained analyst. While we welcome the peculiar strain of psychologically minded clinician who seeks to devote the time, money and mental energy to formal institutional analytic training, we've sent out other invitations to the dinner party. This also caters to mental health professionals who have been practicing for a while; those who have a broad interest in psychoanalysis but aren't especially familiar with specific theoretical details. Maybe a therapist dipped a toe into psychoanalytic theory in graduate school, or maybe they're working through an aversion to it triggered by the sheer mention of Freud's name. No matter if you're leading groups, doing intakes, conducting family therapy, or in individual sessions, it's all fair game – the letters after your name are an afterthought.

This work also is meant for those fresh out of school who might be trying to get a sense of how to be a therapist. There is a truly overwhelming amount of literature for these beginners to reference on their various personal journeys of identity, and from articles to books to supervisors to Twitter accounts, workshops, and peer groups, you "never feel alone in your office" – a dual-edged sword for sure, as your kitchen is full of many cooks.[2] Unfortunately, the opposite is also true; my research indicates that two-year programs with unfulfilling placements often leave many struggling as soon as they graduate. The young therapist is pushed out of the nest to earn their hours but feels lost, afraid, and desperate. Scrambling madly in an attempt to fly on their own, the altruism of the profession is lost in frantic helplessness – like trying to put out intrapsychic fires without knowing if they're a fireman or a sideshow fire-swallower. This is bolstered by insane levels of competition as therapists hop on TikTok and Instagram to build their brands regardless of the potentially complicated ethical implications around confidentiality, integrity, and competency.[3] Like Jung's wounded healer, these therapists have all the passion to help bring understanding to a broken world and none of the tools. Throughout my experience in the analytic world of New York, speaking to supervisors, mental health counselors, social workers, clinical psychologists, etc., one singular problem has emerged. Maybe you know who's portrayed on the website you paid a freelancer to make for you (and believe me, I would know – I've been that very freelancer!). You could know who's speaking in group supervision, when you project an air of confidence in relaying your expertise. But *who are you in the therapy room?* And who do you want to be?

Who this work is for is also influenced by my experience as an analysand. You might notice that throughout this piece, we refer to literature that references the attitudes, workings, and inner life of both the patient and the therapist. And sometimes, literature that references patients will be used to conceive of the psyches of the therapist. This might be one of the most hotly debated notions in this piece, but in a way, these two different models are one and the same. It's one thing to talk about and examine how a specific case unfolds taking into account individual psychologies. But theories are not for the analytic world to implement onto a class of laymen they seek to help as if their own psychic functions are either a completely private matter or to be used only in an expressly and strategically educational way as they emerge in the countertransference. In some cases (ideally, in many cases) the therapist has even been the patient – perhaps even a patient that was the subject of a paper.[4] When it comes to roles in the session, therapists have a great responsibility on their shoulders to uphold the frame and aid in the patient's self-discovery. But in the few solitary moments in this piece in which we frolic in the realm of the mind, we do not talk of patients or therapists, clients, or analysts. The realm of the mind is an equalizing force. We will indeed talk about roles and how they play out. But we also will talk about people who, fundamentally, are more similar than they are different.

In conclusion, think of the performance therapist here as an all-encompassing term, one for those who seek to practice by a certain doctrine; social workers, mental health counselors, behavioral coaches, doctors of philosophy, and doctors of the medical sort. If any of you, dear reader, have leanings towards seeing patients in even a semi-psychodynamic frame, this work should speak to you, and in turn, you to it. There are bits and pieces here for the analytic novice as much as the analytic expert, and those who know very well their own ability to perform are just as welcome as those who have never once thought about it. The only real goal here is to sow the seeds of curiosity and begin to poke at this strange notion of identity, whatever it may be.

Notes

1 Kernberg et al. (1997). *Psychoanalysis in America: An interview for multi-media encyclopedia of philosophical sciences by RAI.* Milan, Italy: Italian Paths of Culture. Web.
2 IPA, Off the Couch. "Episode 111: The Psychoanalytic Consultant with Glen Gabbard, MD." *International Psychoanalytical Association,* 22 May 2022, https://ipaoffthecouch.org/2022/05/22/episode-111-the-psychoanalytic-consultant-with-glen-gabbard-md/.
3 White, E., & Hanley, T. (2022). Therapist + Social Media = Mental health influencer? Considering the research focusing upon key ethical issues around the use of social media by therapists. *Counselling and Psychotherapy Research,* 1–5. Web.
4 Berman, E. (1995). On Analyzing Colleagues. *Contemporary Psychoanalysis,* 31:521. Web.

Part I

Performance art

Welcome – now, let's get started with a little performance art. *Performance* art, we specify, not *performing* art. The latter is comprised of modalities including singing, acting, music, painting, and other traditional art forms. The former is a different creation entirely which we'll dissect in the coming pages. It's imperative that before we begin talking about how performance art can be used as a tool to examine psychoanalytic identity, we should define the thing first. Its history informs our very discussion here, and its structure creates the building blocks for how therapeutic identity is cultivated. But we don't yet know what it is – so we should find out.

A quick disclaimer (applicable for most sections in this work, in fact) is the following: this is not meant to be an exhaustive chronicle of performance art's history. We have a modest goal here, which is to gain a rough sense of the mythos and leitmotifs fueling the underlying thesis. And to achieve that goal, we begin with a vague idea of how these facets have played out in the world outside of the analytical frame. To exhaustively pace through the annals of performance art history would ultimately be unhelpful in terms of directing attention away from the original argument, which focuses predominantly on psychoanalysis. And frankly, the wonderful thing about performance art is that you needn't be a learned scholar to appreciate its beauty and make it your own. In stark contrast to other forms of art that necessitate years of intense training to execute to the fullest extent of one's ability, performance art is a bit of an enigma – anybody can do it with little to no experience.

Because the requirements are so limited, it stands to reason that if a performance artist doesn't even need to be a scholar in their own field, the same can be said for a performance therapist. To co-opt and tinker with this identity, we only need to understand its roots. Therefore, there are only a few main themes to keep in mind during the segment ahead: *who the performance artist is, how they do what they do,* and *how psychoanalysis views performance art.*

To start, we'll go about learning who the performance artist is by surveying a brief history of the medium. This will provide us with a bit of context for the rest of our study. Next, we'll learn why the performance artist does what they do. We'll examine the state of modern performance art,

DOI: 10.4324/9781003412694-2

conceptions or biases about it all, and some of how the performance artist does what they do. And finally, we'll accomplish our goal of transitioning into a psychological headspace by viewing the crossover of performance art and psychoanalytic thought. This will be another light literature review, something we should become accustomed to throughout the work. The first two notions feed into the third – only by knowing performance art can we consider how it's been understood (or misunderstood) by the psychoanalytic world thus far. Hopefully, that doesn't sound too daunting. *Alors, allons-y.*

Chapter 1

History of performance art

Performance art, the ever-elusive beast, "defies precise or easy definition beyond the simple declaration that it is live performance by artists" – though wouldn't that make things so easy if the definition was that simple (Goldberg, 2011). While the performer of the artwork is the artist, they are not performing in a play or a film. The actor or character does not work within a conventional narrative format, nor a conventional time frame. The performance can be any size in length or scope, planned or unplanned, rehearsed or unrehearsed. In a way, Goldberg says in her definitive work on the history of performance art, "definition would immediately negate the possibility of performance itself" – and so we've got to be content with a definition more ambiguous than most other traditional forms of art (2011).

The performance artist's preference to engage with a nebulous and incomprehensible form of expression is a portrait painted against a complicated background. The establishment of performance art came from a dissatisfaction with the available modes of artistic expression. Rather than conforming to elements artists felt unjustly represented their needs, such as visual art, spoken words, or stage performance, they instead discovered new ways to communicate how they felt. Their bodies became the canvases, their noises became words, and their actions became theater. Simply put, performance art consistently reflected the chaos of the world around it in the only way that felt commensurate: a chaotic way.

The term "performance art" came into popularity in the 1970s, but prior to that, various forms of experimental art served as the groundwork for what we know today. In yet another mixed metaphor, we can just say: the uptown express performance art train stopped first at fiery Futurism and absurdist Dadaism in Europe's 1900s to 1920s, then jetted to Surrealism and American variations from the 1920s to 1950s, and finally, pulled into the station of campy yet insightful Living Art and Post-Modernity, which peaked in the public consciousness from the 1960s to 1980s (Goldberg, 2011). If you'd like to ride the local train instead, the route is much more scenic, passing by stops like "noise music" (Klett & Gerber, 2014), German Bauhaus theater workshops or Black Mountain College (Ellert, 1972), and the rise of "body art"

DOI: 10.4324/9781003412694-3

in the 1970s (Jones, 1998), to name a few. But here, we're going to go over the express roadmap instead.

Our first stop, Futurism, is punctuated by a new slew of wild personalities operating in seedy bars and underground clubs all over Europe. In particular, two that made their mark in both writing and performance are Filippo Marinetti, and later, Dadaist Hugo Ball. As Marinetti is considered something like the father of Futurism, we'll start with him.

A self-proclaimed fascist who authored the fundamental Italian text on fascism, Marinetti was a Futurist for life. Marinetti's first manifesto, the *Manifesto del Futurismo,* ignited the intellectuals of Europe, and sought to free Italy from the perils of its past turmoil of violence, war, and fascism. Bored of the slow, stuffy, lackadaisical and laid-back attitude of his home country, Marinetti's artwork was fixated around his love of speed and movement. He referred to poetry as a "violent attack", and war as "the world's only hygiene" (Marinetti, 1909). In his manifesto, he laid out the goals of the Futurists: to "demolish museums and libraries, fight morality," and bring about a "revolution of fire and passion" (1909). Often, he enjoyed metaphors about art as food; his most famous work, 1932s *The Futurist Cookbook,* is full of statements on art in the satirical style of recipes and etiquette recommendations. To Marinetti, pasta was "passéist," and the first course of every meal should be an egg-shaped piece of ice slathered in chestnut paste. While he never called himself a performance artist specifically, his perspectives lay the groundwork for the years of obscure art yet to come. Though his first works shook up the art world, Marinetti continued to refine his revolution, and over the course of his career, he laid out the primary methodology of performance art, something that carries through to this day: how and why to declaim. Declaiming, to Marinetti, was meant to "liberate intellectuals from the old, static, pacifistic and nostalgic declamation" – a fresh soap box to hop on and speak a new form of truth (Marinetti, 1916). And even now, the performance artist is a declaimer, one who comes in to inject a dose of vitality into what they view as a stale, lackluster culture stuck in antiquated ways of thinking. And so, we're on our way to answering our first question: who is the performance artist? They are a *declaimer.*

In Futurism, the first iteration of performance art was split into categories rather than the current intermingling of art forms we have today, and it sought to subvert preexisting performances like dance, theater, poetry, and music. Marinetti and his cohort had a more political angle than Ball and the Dadaists given the discombobulation of the Italian government in his era. Consequently, and their version of performance art sometimes came in the form of ill-received, scandalous plays akin to a political parody on Saturday Night Live, or "sound poems" like *Battaglia, Peso + Odore,* focused on the sounds, sights, and smells of war.

Hugo Ball, another poet, writer, and performer, wrote his version of an avant-garde call to arms, the Dada Manifesto, in 1916; his drive towards something new and exciting was comparable to Marinetti's, but with a markedly less politicized bent. In defiance against a society desperately trying to resume normalcy after the destruction of World War I, Ball's manifesto, and consequently his work, embraced nonsensical madness, art that had never yet been conceptualized, art that reflected the frayed, absurd state of the world around him.

The Dada Manifesto states that the artist does not "want words that other people have invented ... I want my own stuff, my own rhythm, and vowels and consonants too" (Ball & Pinoncelli, 1916). And even more to the point, in Ball's poem Karawane, which he performed in a costume made entirely of paper, he states, "blago bung blago bung/bosso fataka/ü üü ü!" (Ball, 1917). Whatever commentary any present historian, artist or critic presently feels compelled to transpose on this kind of art, Ball's intent, as indicated in his own manifesto, is clear. Whatever emotion or thought this is attempting to fully embody in verbiage and form is anti-intellectual, anti-establishment, anti-language, anti-everything – anti-art, but pro-expression. And here we have another answer to our question: who is the performance artist? They are *pro-expression*.

This is where we see the beginnings of dadaism form. Tristan Tzara, another eccentric staple of the Cabaret Voltaire and on-again-off-again friend of Ball's, also had a profound impact in formulating Dadaism. Though ridiculous in nature, Tzara said, Dadaism should absolutely be considered a movement within the art community rather than anti-art. In his own manifesto, Tzara put it just as frankly: "Dada was born of a need for independence, of a distrust toward unity"; it is the "abolition of logic;" it is "every object, all objects, sentiments, obscurities, apparitions" engaged in "a protest with the fists of its whole being engaged in destructive action" (Tzara, 1918).

But in the anger of Dadaism, in its rejection of society's hypocritical value system, artists sought to create something for themselves, something free, something without duplicity and hollowness. Whereas the Futurists aspired to cleanse the world with screaming fire and brimstone, the Dadaists simply wanted to scream, even if it was just for the sake of screaming – with humor and autonomy, with whimsy and emotion, with natural off-the-cuff flow and unrelenting confusion. And if the rest of the world would call it art, as they did with vibrancy, excitement, and whole-heartedness, all the better for them. Unfortunately for the Dadaists, initially, they did not, and Dadaists were seen as grotesque and vile contrarians making a mockery of the once-sacred notion of art.

As the years went by, performance art eventually found a happy medium in between irrationality and meaning. While political statements have always been at the core of many performance artist's goals, those goals also manifested over the years in slightly softer social statements, personal statements, or even absurdist statements. It is neither about one very particular thing, nor nothing at all; oftentimes, performance art is about everything, as can be seen in its evolution. Whereas performance art formally began with Ball and his Cabaret Voltaire pals in Zurich dressing in costumes and reading out sound poems, over the course of half a century, the public was soon inundated with abstract expressions fitting perfectly with the dissonance of their respective eras.

To each decade of society, there was an anti-society; to each decade of art, there was an anti-art. Various John Cages and Jackson Pollacks first began stunning audiences and curators around the world with art that only barely resembled its predecessors. And once the bizarre became cutting-edge, performance art began to work its way into the mainstream, appreciated by artists and chichi art lovers alike. The 1960s and 1970s saw performance art come alive as sub-movements began to form, from the Gutai in Japan (Tiampo, 2011) to The Living Theater in New York City, or even the controversial and grotesque Wiener Aktionismus in Vienna (Schmatz & Daniel, 1992). In Carol Schneeman's "action painting" as she hung from a tree (1976), art became known as something more than just acrylics on a canvas or music in a symphony hall. Just as art became pro-expression when the Dadaists turned words into sounds, it became pro-self as Living Artists turned their bodies into canvases. And we have another answer: who is the performance artist? They are *pro-self*.

Through the 1980s all the way to the present day, many of these artists have maintained a level of popularity, especially among both persistently frustrated, untrained youths and highly educated post-modern artists and art lovers. Works like Nam June Paik's stacked televisions at the Whitney (1989; Smith, 2019) showed that the days of art as a pedestalized and classical fixture were over. The general public was now able to reach out and touch an artist, "to be a spectator of its ritual and its distinct community, and to be surprised by the unexpected, always unorthodox presentations that the artists devise" (Goldberg, 2011). And as performance art has become more accessible than ever, the performance artist becomes a voice for the people like never before. Marina Abramović is still communing intimately with strangers for hours at a time (2010), Laurie Anderson is still winning Grammy's for experimental music about natural disasters (Hill, 2019), and Yoko Ono is still screaming at the top of her lungs into microphones at the MoMA in New York (Rosenberg, 2010), all in the name of art.

With the advent of the internet, up-and-coming performance artists can show their material to the world through sites like YouTube, a new underground Zurich cabaret in its own right, as they make their own grassroots efforts at insight and success. As early theory affirmed that Dadaists "recognize no theory" (Tzara, 1918), untrained performers completely unknown in the formal art world, like the avantgarde pioneer Emilia Fart, garner over a million views with achievements such as "Why I dress like an obese, deranged Judge Judy" (2017). They can also be found, like the wealthy institution of Banksy does, making a performative commentary by destroying their own art just minutes after it's sold, in an attempt at offending the likewise wealthy institution of art dealing (Daley, 2018). Musical artists, who formerly stayed within the bounds of their field, feel the freedom to expand their artistic purvey. The incomparable Lady Gaga tells the world, "I consider myself to be a performance artist. ... My whole life is performance" – and much like many celebrities these days, "every time she appears in public—even just walking down the street—she is performing" (Benton, 2010). One could even argue that obligatorily performance as a character in the public eye, for the sake of yourself or to raise awareness for a larger moral or ethical concern, transforms the performer's life into art; anyone from Andy Kaufman to Kim Kardashian, or even Hillary Clinton, who read her personal emails at a performance art festival in Venice might agree (Mansoor, 2019). And so we have our final answer: who is the performance artist? They are all of us.

References

Goldberg, R.L. (2011). *Performance art: From futurism to the present* (Rev. and enl.). H.N. Abrams. Web.

Klett, J., & Gerber, A. (2014). The meaning of indeterminacy: Noise music as performance. *Cultural Sociology, 8*(3), 275–290. Web. 10.1177/1749975514523936

Ellert, J. (1972). The bauhaus and black mountain college. *The Journal of General Education, 24*(3), 144–152. Web.

Jones, A. (1998). *Body art/performing the Subject.* Minneapolis, MN: University of Minnesota Press. Print.

Marinetti, F.T. (1909). The futurist manifesto. *Le Figaro, 51*(20), 39–44. Web.

Marinetti, F.T., & Flint, R.W. (1916/1972). *Marinetti: Selected writings.* New York: Farrar, Straus and Giroux.

Ball, H., & Pinoncelli, P. (Eds.). (1916). *Le manifeste dada (the dada manifesto).* Saint-Étienne, France: Le Réalgar. Web.

Ball, H. (1917). Karawane. *Dada Almanach.* Zurich, Switzerland: Erich Reiss. Web.

Tzara, T. (1918). *Dada manifesto.* Zurich, Switzerland: Cabaret Voltaire. Web.

Tiampo, M. (2011). *Gutai: Decentering modernism.* Chicago, IL: University of Chicago Press. Print.

Schmatz, F., & Daniel, J. (1992). Viennese actionism and the Vienna group: The Austrian Avant-Garde after 1945. *Discourse, 14*(2), 59–73.

Paik. (1989). *Fin de siecle II [performance].* New York: Whitney Museum of American Art.

Smith, R. (2019). *Nam June Paik at the Whitney: A work of dizzying complexity.* New York: The New York Times. Web.

Schneemann, C. (1976). *Up to and including her limits.* Madrid: Museo Nacional Centro Reina Sofia.

Abramović, M. (2010). *The artist is present.* New York: MoMA. Web.

Hill, M. (2019). *Punch brothers, Laurie Anderson, Kronos Quartet win Grammy awards.* New York: Nonesuch. Web.

Rosenberg, K. (2010). *Commentary that's both visual and vocal.* New York: The New York Times. Web.

Fart, E. (Director). (2017, Nov 19). [Internet] *Why I dress like an obese, deranged Judge Judy*. Montreal, Canada.

Daley, J. (2018). Watch this $1.4 million Banksy painting shred itself as soon as it's sold. *Smithsonian Magazine*. Washington, DC: Smithsonian Institute. Web.

Benton, R.J. (2010). Lady Gaga's Penis. *Psychoanalytic Perspectives*, 7(2): 297–317. Web.

Mansoor, S. (2019). *Hillary Clinton reads controversial emails at Italian art show*. New York: Time Magazine. Web.

Chapter 2

Performance art in practice

Now, we talk about how the performance artist performs. How they look in the wild, were you to pass one on the street. A pro-expression, pro-self declaimer – the everyman. Much like the Dadaists were misunderstood because their stylings were so bizarre, modern conceptions of performance art can sometimes vary from the artist's intent (if there is any intent in the work to begin with). What performance artists are truly doing in their work is important to think about when building a foundation of knowledge concerning this field. And the literature on performance art, as any literature that rears its little head in the distanced world of academia, can very much differ from the practice. This is especially the case in modernity, when some performance artists are not well aware of the history behind the medium, as the medium is meant for the everyman. Thus, to determine what the performance artist does, we must look for patterns – both in the performance art of yore and in the performance art of the present.

The first and most well-known reason a performance artist performs is to *shock*. One could say that the goal is to shock audiences, but among performance artists, that notion is split. Some believe that audiences are integral to performance art and the work wouldn't exist without them, others say that they're just a secondary factor in the piece (Ward, 2012). Performance art to this day remains a staple of awe and disgust, just like the leading lady from John Water's *Female Trouble,* Dawn Davenport, would want it. Some even elicit discomfort without an end-goal or product in mind other than "shocking audiences into reassessing their own notions of art and its relation to culture" (Goldberg, 2011). Like a chaotic modern version of Futurists, they perpetrate chaos for its own sake. Performance art has skyrocketed in intensity – no longer yelling vowels on a dimly lit cabaret stage, they now participate in self-immolation – not for the sake of a political statement, but to astonish judges on America's Got Talent. As declaimers, performance artists screech and holler, flail and wail, decry and denounce in whatever language might best suit their message. All in the name of art, or anti-art.

Why performance artists love to shock varies from person to person. Bodies are put on the line, sliced and diced like so many cured meats on a

DOI: 10.4324/9781003412694-4

charcuterie board. Chris Burden was shot on video (1971) and crucified on a blue Volkswagen Beetle (1974) (a busy few years!) – Mao Sugiyama's piece *Testicle Banquet* involved the cooking and eating of his own genitalia (2012). Performance artist Orlan underwent a series of plastic surgeries on video (including various head implants) and Hermann Nitsch has been performing animal sacrifices in the name of art for decades, much to the disgust of audiences. Lai Thi Dieu Ha ironed pig bladders (2010) and Deborah de Robertis displayed her own *Origin of the World* (namely, her vagina) in front of Courbert's actual *Origin of the World* (2014). And while these artists would certainly argue that their shocking performances have hidden meanings, they turn a layman's conception of modern performance art into "a funny kind of catchall, deployed to imbue something with high-art pretension, or to explain work that's otherwise inexplicable" (Petrusich, 2018).

But the performance artist isn't just one who participates in grotesque or outlandish acts. What they do can also be mundanely asinine. George Brecht of Fluxus, a group from the 1960s, wrote "event scores;" "simple instructions to complete everyday tasks," such as the Three Chair Event, in which – you guessed it! – a participant sits in a black chair, then a yellow chair, and finally a white chair (Wood, 2015). And just a few short years ago, we have bananas being taped to a wall by one performance artist, just to be eaten whole by another (Elassar, 2019). Each action is labeled as art, justified as an iconic cultural moment by one side of the media, and mocked as the epitome of stupidity by the other (White, 2016). "Half the people thought I'm an idiot who just eats a banana," Datuna the banana-eater said at his own gallery opening in Chelsea, "but the other half got it" (Bashura, 2020).

While the gruesome factor may be significantly lower in a performance art piece about fruit, the question of intent, meaning, and interpretation still remain. Ultimately, Datuna may have the right idea. What a performance artist does is they shock. But they don't just shock with the intention of causing their audience to recoil. They provide a shock to the system – any system – that has been functioning in the status quo for too long. They provide a shock that allows viewers to question what they know and why they might think they know it. It shocks one out of an old, stale way of declaiming, just as Marinetti says. And whether it makes people enraged, fascinated, thrilled, or nonplussed, it makes them feel something. And what is a performance art piece if not a tool for thinking and feeling?

Another thing the performance artist can do is that by becoming the everyman, they *engage* with whoever might be listening, allowing everyone around them to become their critics. These days, performance art is commonly interpreted by the public eye through the self-involved, experimental lenses of both our current Westernized sociocultural views and technology-fueled inclinations to already pre-existing narcissistic tendencies (Bucknell, 2017; White, 2016). It is no longer an underground movement, but a very visible one, subject to scrutiny not just from the cultural elite, but from anyone, whether they're a world-renowned art critic or JC Penney cashier. Whether one's retrospective at the Guggenheim just premiered or they're bemoaning the genre of music in a bar, everybody's got something to say. But in many ways, this is one of the long-embattled goals of performance art: to reach the layman and make them reconsider some of their beliefs. Performance art of yore was often presented as introspective works performed with impunity, so ludicrous that any public scrutiny was not only welcome but anticipated. It analyzed oneself in the world or one's experience of justice, integrity, or society, with the person performing the art almost as an inconsequential modality to transport the message. And now, because performance artworks usually have no script, "the reader is at the mercy of the critic, dependent on him not only for an analysis and evaluation of the work but also for the description upon which his judgments are based" (Mehta, 1990). Getting anyone and everyone involved in an emotional way is almost a necessity for these works to become engrained into culture.

Another one of the most misunderstood things about a performance artist is the way they can express the desire to be *pro-self*. Engaging and shocking viewers also means attracting attention to themselves. Whether performance artists are performing something or they are the artwork themselves, to some of the aforementioned critics, their involvement centralizes the performer rather than the performance. It becomes less about the message and more about the medium – *'look at me, ma, I'm avant-garde!'* But being pro-self doesn't automatically mean being self-obsessed or self-focused. In some ways, and for some performers, the self is used as a tool to best relay the message of the artwork, whether that message best corresponds to a corporeal, spiritual, emotional, athletic, or other medium – like an artist choosing a canvas over a guitar. Does a painting centralize the canvas or the picture; does a song centralize the instruments or the music? Deconstructing the haughty artist and their haughty self-image, the performance artist's body is the medium and the world is the message, though it might be difficult to separate the two at times. And to them, being pro-self means using one's whole being to embody the quiddity of their artistic beliefs. So, while in some ways the performance artist makes the self a necessity for the work to occur, they also make the self an afterthought – something used as a tool, but not the only tool, to complete the artwork.

In the tradition of Marinetti, today, we have been talking about and will continue to talk about food. To capture what the performance artist does, consider this metaphor. The performance artist sees the world like a plate of raw carrots; they take it in, digest it, and as the proteins and vitamins seep into their bloodstream and combine with their own very individualized biochemical makeup, it changes them as they embody the structure. It is a part of them but is ultimately produced by an item they ingested; carrots, geopolitical stresses,[1] al frescoes of John F. Kennedy's assassination, or any other stimuli the world can offer. One takes in experiences, and spits them out; one ingests stimuli, and gives it back to the world in the only way they knew how to process it. If that doesn't sound familiar yet, don't fret – it will soon.

Note

1   See Introduction.

References

Goldberg, R.L. (2011). *Performance art: From futurism to the present* (Rev. and enl.). H.N. Abrams. Web.

Ward, F. (2012). *No innocent bystanders: Performance art and audience*. Dartmouth, MA, USA: Dartmouth College Press.

Burden, C. (1971). *Shoot [performance]*. Santa Ana, CA: F Space Gallery.

Burden, C. (1974). *Trans-Fixed [performance]*. Venice, CA.

Sugiyama, M. (2012). *Testicle Banquet [performance]*. Tokyo, Japan.

Bucknell, A. (2017). Can anything be performance art? *Artsy*. New York: Artsy. Web.

Mehta, X. (1990). Performance art: Problems with description and evaulation. *Journal of Dramatic Theory and Criticism*, 5(1), 187–199.

White, B. (2016). 'Performance art' as pejorative. *The Awl*. New York. Web.

Ha, L.D. (2010). *Fly Off [performance]*. Hanoi, Vietnam: Nha San Studio.

de Robertis, D. (2014). *Origin of the World [performance]*. Paris, France: Musée d'Orsay.

Petrusich, A. (2018). *Why are pop stars trying to be performance artists?* New York: The New Yorker. Web.

Wood, A. (2015). *Performance art*. New York: Gareth Stevens Publications.

Elassar, A. (2019). Man who ate the $120,000 banana art installation says he isn't sorry and did it to create art. *CNN*. New York: Warner Media. Web.

Bashura, H. (2020). The artist who ate the art basel banana returns with a surprisingly sentimental exhibition of his own. *Hyperallergic*. Brooklyn, NY: Newspack. Web.

Chapter 3

Performance art in psychoanalysis

In the last appetizer in our performance art course, we'll look at how performance art is seen through the eyes of psychoanalysis, which has long held an affair with the artistic realm in general. The relationship is filled with quixotic case studies and impassioned musings on the way that visual and performing arts can be examined through the analytic frame. Books praise the artwork of obscure painters as unconscious masterpieces, id-driven dances are evaluated with intellectual intensity, and even pop star Lady Gaga is analyzed as a "powerful, phallic woman" (Benton, 2010). But rather than delving into the world of analysis and art, which is a field all on its own, we're looking to contextualize analysis in a different medium: that of performance art, one cohesive element, with one cohesive definition that we've just been over ad-nauseum. And as we said before, performance art isn't strictly an art – sometimes, it can be an anti-art, or art-averse. But does psychoanalysis see it in the way we've defined it? Or do they see it in another way?

What is performance art to psychoanalysis?

Psychoanalysis views performance art in a fashion that's sometimes laden with misunderstandings – and understandably so. On the surface, the fields of psychoanalysis and performance art may not appear to be well-fitting puzzle pieces –while many are taught that analysis is like an ancient tongue, performance art by nature has no language, rejecting these "words that other people have invented" (Ball & Pinoncelli, 1916). Psychoanalysis is a world of particular rules; performance art was made directly in opposition of rules. Psychoanalysis is very particular with technique; performance art is a mockery of technique. And performance art can sometimes be either a metaphor, simile, or euphemism for an artistic brand of neuroticism that's expressed in a nonsensical way.

Unfortunately for us, these examinations are more about the act of performance (insofar as an actor would perform in a play) than performance art itself. Consequently, we'll have to be a little picky during this meal and reserve

DOI: 10.4324/9781003412694-5

our appetites for the latter rather than the former. One must not forget that performance art is supposed to be something outside the realm of traditional art – so much so that it bucks the traditions of pens to paper, paintbrushes to canvases, and actors to the stage. Performance art, one term with one meaning, is not a "performing art" per se, though it can be. A computer programmer can be a performance artist as much as any dancer or painter could. So, while a therapist might have an artistic lens when they're examining their own technique, as previously mentioned, we will hesitate to generalize psychotherapy as an art as much as we'll shy away from calling it a science.

In the literature, performance art is also conflated with "performative," a concept popularized by gender theorist Judith Butler, but were used before her to talk about performance in speech (Austin, 1975; Derrida, 1972). While performativity originally was meant to describe the ways in which individuals act out perceived gender norms, it was then extrapolated to mean any sort of performance of the self that inauthentically exaggerates characteristics as a means to some kind of social end (Butler, 1988). The underlying causes of performativity are complex. In some cases, one may be performative in the attempt to convince another that these traits are a part of their characterological tapestry. Performativity can be a defense against being seen a certain way – attempting to be seen in a certain way, perhaps as a positive person or a carefree person (Atsalis, 2011). One could also be performative satirically and intentionally, putting on a sort of show for their adoring public (Lloyd, 1999). One who dresses in expensive outfits to put on an air of wealth is considered performative. Another feature of performativity is that the performer continues to engage in it regardless as to if this ruse is transparent to others or not – and no matter who contests their behavior, the performer will defend their act to the last.

Though performance art can be performative to serve a greater purpose (for hyperbolic effect, social commentary, or shock value), it does not always need to be performative (as we spoke about in the more mundane, banana-eating forms of performance art). Psychoanalysis, interestingly, is the same way; flashy interpretations and Academy Award-winning scenes aren't a part of every session. The main difference between performance and performativity is just that: a performance is something between two people, something that can be relatively tame and exist in many forms. And being performative is something that happens with one person, where their idea of a feature is exaggerated due to the internal machinations of their own intrapsychic world. And in the realm of psychoanalytic literature on performance art, we have both in spades.

How is it written about?

Psychoanalytic literature about performance art takes a few forms. Theorists have picked apart how the actual space of the therapeutic frame can provide for a kind of performance (for instance, the enactments and dances in a sort of psychic realm so beautifully outlined in Aron's Dramatic Dialogues (2016)). Often, the metaphysical play enacted between the analyst and patient is at the center of these explorations of analysis and performance art. Performances are linked to myth, ritual, and phantasies – they are considered by some to be an enactment of the primal scene, filled with tragedy and oedipal longing (Arvanitakis, 1998). The dyad of patient and therapist are sometimes compared to actors in a play, reciting lines both literal and metaphorical written by the patient. In this way, the performance occurs in a liminal psychic space rather than a visible roleplay.

Let's begin with "performance art" or "performance artist" from the perspective of the patients. The term is used almost flippantly sometimes as a bit of a catch-all for someone engaging in something that seems like a performing art in its expression (which, if we recall, is a bit of a misnomer). Performance art takes on connotations of falseness displayed both consciously and unconsciously (Chaplan, 2013), sublimation, and grandiosity (Axelrod, 1994). We have serious mental illness being thought of as a sort of performance art (Campoli, 2019) alongside suicide (Chassay, 2006) and narcissism (Giesbrecht, 2003). Both idolized as the ultimate artistic achievement and demonized as an act of fakeness or self-involvement, performance art is utilized by the analytic world like anything else is: as a tool for understanding a patient. But the therapist is rarely examined as a performance artist – only as a "performer."

The literature on a therapist as a performer is rich, and doesn't discriminate; therapists are compared to musicians, painters, sculptors, and of course, stage performers. Performance as a therapist is about the practitioner as an actor, a topic many an actor-turned-therapist are happy to analyze, consider, and teach (O'Connell, 2019). Some therapists also live double lives as artists on the side, and to them, writing, painting, photography, acting, and singing all inform their perspectives (Urdang, 2018). Like the artist, Beres says, "the psychoanalyst shares with the artist the search for inner thoughts and feelings" – but the therapist's technique brings the unconscious content of the patient to the surface while someone like a poet, working alone, allows the content to surface in whatever way it might unintentionally (1981).

Rarely, however, are therapists compared to performance artists, other than by a select few. Therapists like Kavanaugh (2010) states that psychoanalysis functions as a performance art as it reflects interpersonal and psychic truths – much like surrealist Antonin Artaud's *Theatre of Cruelty* (1958) in which one's perception of themselves is dissolved through unnerving, fiery performance. Its passionate, rigorous, painful, and enlightening nature, Kavanaugh says, is meant to "speak with the more barbaric, primitive, and real aspects of self and other." The performance of a patient crying (sometimes loudly or fervently) can create a catharsis – the performance of a patient yelling can lead to an understanding about their anger. This isn't an act, as this behavior is real and comes from a place of true hurt. But the presentation, in all its intensity, reflects the psychic reality of the patient in a way that elicits the same horrific, grotesque shock of a Viennese Actionist urinating into their comrade's mouth on a stage (Sheik, 2020).

Alan Karbelnig has done far and above the most extensive writing on viewing the therapist themselves as a kind of performance artist. To Karbelnig, the comparison begins because the therapist consistently integrates elements like "morals, aesthetic sensibilities, imaginativeness, and originality" into their work like a performance artist does (2016b). He even says that there's an element of improvisation in psychoanalysis, as a therapist has got to say the right thing on the fly. Just as an actor or singer would describe their body as an instrument of art, Karbelnig says that therapists "deliver their framing, presence, and engagement services" to patients and clients using only themselves (2016a). To Karbelnig, each performance is special and individualized, as each performance artist is "shaped by biology, history, and culture, as well as through their immediate life experiences" (2016b). There is even more at play – the therapist's morals and values, their sense of aesthetics (how they decorate their offices and their bodies as therapists), and their respective imaginations and originality.

In the world of performance, Karbelnig says, these three elements are crucial: *framing* is the creation of the space, *presence* is the investment that both the performer and audience have in their performance, and *engagement* describes how the involvement of all parties involved (2014). This is then translated into the format of therapy: framing is the office and way your practice operates, presence is the mental bandwidth both the patient and the therapist are bringing to the session, and engagement are the words that flow from each.

Our friend performativity also has a special place in the literature, and while many papers are on Butler's popular gender performativity concept, some theorists have taken the idea of performativity and extended it to other realms. The analytic "language," as it were, meaning the verbal and non-verbals methods that the unconscious communicates in the analytic space, actually also underwent a bit of a crisis of performativity (Green, 2002). Analytic speech is bound by desire and transference, he says, and any professional or theoretical attempt to talk around the issues end up as a kind of performative prudishness. Harris argues that performativity can become consciously or unconsciously ironic, as self-states frequently shift and the therapist ends up trying a bit too hard to convey a feeling that's felt quite simply (2005).

And that's about where the current literature of performance art and psychoanalysis ends. We have some books on performance art as a method of art therapy, clinicians placing a psychoanalytic lens on performance art, and a twelve-course meal of books on art and psychoanalysis. And as any researcher could tell you, I'm sure there's some odds and ends missing that will make it into future editions of this book. Ultimately, the thing we can learn from this section is as follows: performance art is mostly seen by the psychoanalytic community within the literature *as just another art form* rather than an embodiment of a belief or form using a certain kind of personalized expression. From these perspectives, it *is* expressly art rather than art-adjacent, and often indicates a kind of romanticized action that both indicates and serves as an attempt to conceal a deeper feeling beneath.

However, "mostly" does not cover it all. A few select theorists see performance art as more than just another esoteric artistic concept to contemplate with feigned depth. The analyst has been examined as a performance artist before – this idea is not new. To Karbelnig, performance art comes out in the very ways the therapist acts, existing in a tangible realm outside that of the more abstract intellectual sphere. To Kavanaugh, the deepest most carnal parts of the id are the true performance, eschewing "words other people have invented" for a more expressive and emotional kind of language (Ball & Pinoncelli, 1916). And to Atwood (2010), performance art is constantly "expressing to the world an indomitable life spirit within," a spirit that is both stalwart and powerful – but nothing more specific than a reflection of the inner self. And this is exactly where therapy rests; not fully an art but also not fully a science, it rather seeks to externalize the internal processes of all things in an attempt to understand them.

This is the aim of the performance therapist. In order for them to symbolize their own personalized impressions of theory, they must be able to grasp what performance means to them insofar as how they present, act, and choose to be – just as one must recognize what art means to them in order to choose how they subvert it. But defining performance is no easy undertaking. In order to do so, this therapist, no matter what theoretical perspective they most adore, must begin to examine their own identities – perhaps in a different way than ever before.

References

Benton, R.J. (2010). Lady Gaga's Penis. *Psychoanalytic Perspectives, 7*(2), 297–317. Web.

Ball, H., & Pinoncelli, P. (Eds.). (1916). *Le manifeste dada (the dada manifesto)*. Saint-Étienne, France: Le Réalgar. Web.

Derrida, J. (1972). Signature event context. In S. Weber & J. Mehlman trans., *Limited Inc* (pp. 1–23). Evanston: Northwestern University Press.

Austin, J.L., & Urmson, J.O. (1975). *How to Do Things with Words*. Harvard University Press.

Butler, J. (1988). Performative acts and gender constitution: An essay in phenomenology and feminist theory. *Theatre Journal, 40*(4), p. 519.

Atsalis, E. (2011). Emotion: New psychosocial perspectives. S. Day-Sclater, D. W. Jones, H. Price, & C. Yates (eds.), *Organizational and Social Dynamics* (11, pp. 121–127). London: Palgrave Macmillan.

Lloyd, M. (1999). Performativity, parody, politics. *Theory, culture & society, 16*(2), 195–213.

Arvanitakis, K.I. (1998). A theory of theater: Theater as theory. *Psychoanalysis and Contemporary Thought, 21*, 33–60.

Aron, L., & Atlas, G. (2016). Dramatic dialogue: Dreaming & drama in contemporary clinical practice. *Psychoanalytic Perspectives, 16*, 249–271.

Chaplan, R. (2013). How to help get stuck analyses unstuck. *Journal of the American Psychoanalytic Association, 61*, 591–604.

Axelrod, S.D. (1994). "Impossible projects": Men's illusory solutions to the problem of work. *Psychoanalytic Psychology 11*:21–32.

Campoli, G. Ed., Lombardi R., Rinaldi L., & Thanopulos S. (2019). Psychoanalysis of the psychoses: Current developments in theory and practice. *International Journal of Psychoanalysis, 100*, 428–432.

Chassay, S. (2006). Death in the afternoon. *International Journal of Psychoanalysis, 87*, 203–217.

Urdang, E. (2018). Art, creativity, and psychoanalysis: Perspectives from analyst-artists. In Hagman, G. (ed.), *Psychoanalytic Social Work* (25, pp. 74–78). New York: Routledge.

Beres, D. (1981). Self, identity, and narcissism. *Psychoanalytic Quarterly, 50*, 515–534.

O'Connell, M. (2019). *The performing art of therapy: Acting insights and techniques for clinicians* (1st ed.). Abingdon, Oxfordshire, UK: Routledge. 10.4324/9781315175683

Karbelnig, A. (2014). The sanctuary of empathy and the invitation of engagement: Psychic retreat, kafka's A hunger artist, and the psychoanalytic process. *The Psychoanalytic Review, 101*, 895–924.

Karbelnig, A. (2016a). Stirred by Kafka's a country doctor: An exploration of psychoanalysts' styles, vulnerabilities, and surrealistic journeys. *Psychoanalytic Review, 103*, 69–101.

Karbelnig, A. (2016b). "The analyst is present": Viewing the psychoanalytic process as performance art. *Psychoanalytic Psychology, 33*, S153–S172.

Kavanaugh, P.B. (2010). Escaping the phantom's ghostly grasp: On psychoanalysis as a performance art in the spirit world. *Psychoanalytic Review, 97*, 733–756.

Sheik, A. (2020). Visualizing social effects: A Marxist analysis of Hermann Nitsch's 'poured painting': The crucifixion. *South African Journal of Art History, 35*(1). Gale Academic OneFile.

Harris, A. (2005). Conflict in relational treatments. *Psychoanalytic Quarterly, 74*, 267–29.

Atwood, G. (2010). The abyss of madness: An interview. *International Journal of Psychoanalytic Self Psychology, 5*, 334–356.

Giesbrecht, H. (2003). Body art: Narcissism of Eros. *Canadian Journal of Psychoanalysis, 11*, 465–491.

Part II

Identity

Now that we have a semi-firm definition of performance art outlined, we can move onto the next course: performance in the psychoanalytic world. What we're here to do is look at the intersection of psychoanalysis and performance art to conceptualize therapeutic identity, and our abbreviated education in the history of performance art will be complimented here by an abbreviated history of performance in psychoanalysis. But the heading of this section says "Identity," you say, not "Performance"! Don't worry – it will all fall into place.

Preliminarily, this section will outline how performance is conceptualized in the world of psychoanalysis because performance is a way in which identity is expressed. There are a number of interchangeable terms that one can use for the overall authentic identity that meshes with the performance we speak of here – the self, personhood, selfhood, and so on, and so forth. Here, we'll take a broader look at first what "performance" means in psychoanalysis, and then how it relates to the "self" or "identity." Like separating egg whites from their yolks, we will learn what parts of oneself are a performance, what parts are not, and what that means for the individual. And yes, we are indeed working under the notion that performance is inherently part of one's identity – the argument here is that there is an inherent contradiction between one's genuine internal state and their performative self, or the self that one wishes to either communicate or be received as by the surrounding world. Bear with us to learn more about how.

Identity, the self, personhood, and selfhood (or any other synonym you can think of) as far as the therapist is concerned is often less about the intimate details of their intrapsychic workings about the more dichotomous and practical matter of their presentation in session. Colloquially, identity is a somewhat flexible endeavor and dependent on one's situation. In the psychoanalytic world, a widely known conceptualization of the "self" is Bromberg's self-states: how one person can have numerous different ways they appear, act, think, and feel dependent upon the situation they're in (1996). Other less analytic literature has a sort of concrete definition of

DOI: 10.4324/9781003412694-6

identity: a primary self and a second self, in which the former is one's personality and disposition outside of work and the latter is what someone is like at work. The second term for a second self is a "work ego," referenced everywhere from Milgram's studies on behaviors shifting to meet social expectations (1974) to Zimbardo's findings that a uniform can create a persona that's unrecognizable to the person donning the outfit (1973). The conversation around identity as a therapist is about how to be professional, how to maintain boundaries, and how to ethically provide good care in any situation. Even analytic literature can refer to the work ego as more focused, more goal oriented, more empathetic, accepting, and reasonable (Fliess, 1942). Even the least psychologically minded of us can see the merit in this argument; I mind my professionalism at work and don't at home. But what does that *really* mean?

Why learning more about identity feeds into our larger argument of the performance therapist is likewise just as simple. In determining how the therapist comprehends the act of understanding – either the patient or their own countertransference – they can then begin to perform in ways that reflect that understanding. In short, the analyst seeks to aid the patient in understanding themselves. To do that, *they* must understand themselves, making an identity an out of performance, authenticity, constructs, and truths, all whipped into one smooth dish like a sumptuous garlic mashed potato. But this is just a claim – a claim we will now substantiate using psychoanalytic literature.

This leads us to the following sections, where various theories of identity are explored through the eyes of four theorists: Sigmund Freud, Carl Jung, Karen Horney, and D.W. Winnicott. Through these scholars we can gain a greater foundation of how identity is perceived in the realm of psychoanalysis. But much like the history of performance art, this section is merely a sample platter of the many wonderful ways to conceptualize identity – namely, the focus is on the contrast between the outer and the inner, the external-facing and the internal-facing, the way things seem versus the way they might truly be.

Psychoanalysis and the self

As we look at the plate in front of us, with just a glance we can firmly state that this course is a complex one. But other diners do not always see it that way. Often, "performance" in the analytic world is taken literally. We've mentioned how therapists often talk about themselves in the literature as if they're "performing" as actors, musicians, or dancers. But the performance of a therapist – and who they are underneath that performance – is more akin to a state of being rather than the act of stepping on stage. Karbelnig stresses that this necessity for "reactivity, improvisation, and spontaneity" must be present "in order to successfully reach ... the cages in which their patients psychically reside;" so while there aren't lines to be said, or characters to be played, the actual mindful performance the therapist is a vital tool for the patient (2014). It is an overarching idea; a way in which to be, and also a way in which to do. One is not acting like a character when they are a therapist – one *is* a therapist.

This is why performance is inherently a portion of the self (interchangeable here with the terms selfhood, or personhood). Think of performance art as it's been described in prior sections; namely one's ingestion of the metaphorical carrots and the orange hue it creates. And no matter the makeup, long-sleeved shirts, or skin lasering procedures they undergo, they will still be orange. It is an expression of their insides shown on the outside. This is identity: how one takes in, interprets, and expresses the various stimuli in their lives. This continued phenomenon is subjective, as two different people can take in the same experience and turn two completely different shades of orange.

Additionally, this discussion of identity and performance is not factually comparable to the wacky Dadaist creations Cabaret Voltaire. Therapists are (for the most part) not flinging other's carrots around like chefs at a Hibachi grill, waiting for the audience's rapt approval. Instead, this concept is about how the mind structures and equalizes more authentic sections of one's selfhood with more performative ones. These performative elements can be indicative of resolved or unresolved internal conflict, and they can exist in a multitude of theories. And the more one tries to hide them, the more apparent and troublesome they become – as is the case with any seemingly well-structured defense mechanism. Insofar as the therapist is concerned, this conceptualization of identity still stands.

Now that we've explored performance and defined identity, let's begin to pick it apart from a psychoanalytic perspective. The self in relation to the world – whether it's the patient, the analyst, the electrician, barista, football player, politician, or hooker – bends and molds around the situations they find themselves in and the people they find themselves around. We've made that abundantly clear. But the overarching notion of what it means to have a stable "self" despite an ever-changing environment is one of most prolific topics in psychoanalysis. Almost every theorist had a way in which to see the structure of the self, and how these instances of time, place, and social label inform everyone's identities at large. We can imagine how one might begin to think about the therapist's task of understanding it for themselves, as they too have their own impressions of how the human mind is psychically arranged, judging by their own work and study. It's a massive undertaking, we think as we look at our pasta course. However, it's not an impossible one.

What follows are a few forays into some various models of the mind – historically, how psychoanalytic thinkers have structured the self. Some believe that identity is a meshing of inner and outer selves, others believe that identity is composed of multiple parts. Some believe that inauthentic and defensive performances (dare we say, performativity?) are a natural part of identity cultivation, others do not. Let us be reminded that these explorations don't necessarily serve as hard and fast rules for the performing therapist's methodology because we certainly wouldn't want to play into the old stereotype of psychotherapists who overly identify with very specific theoretical orientations. But without an idea of how to conceptualize the self from a psychoanalytic perspective, we won't have any idea of how it's expressed to the world – and consequently, how those two states fit together.

References

Bromberg, P.M. (1996). Standing in the spaces: The multiplicity of self and the psychoanalytic relationship. *Contemporary Psychoanalysis, 32*(4), 509–535. Web.

Milgram, S. (1974). *Obedience to authority: An experimental view*. New York: Harper & Row, 1974.

Zimbardo, P., Banks, C., & Haney, C. (1973). Interpersonal dynamics in a simulated prison. *International Journal of Criminology & Penology, 1*(1), 69–97.

Karbelnig, A. (2014). The sanctuary of empathy and the invitation of engagement: Psychic retreat, kafka's A hunger artist, and the psychoanalytic process. *The Psychoanalytic Review, 101*(6), 895–924.

Fliess, R. (1942). The metapsychology of the analyst. *The Psychoanalytic Quarterly, 11*, 211–227.

Chapter 4

The tripartite structure

The most obvious place to start looking at the self in the world of psychoanalysis would be in the structure of the self-itself: the superego, the id, and ego, all wrapped into one bundle called the *tripartite structure*. Thousands of papers have been written about this topic alone, and this baseline structure is one of the first concepts that any young therapist learns in their extended education. Tripartite itself means "three parts," and the term "tripartite" can also be used colloquially in the psychology world to mean anything with three facets. Interestingly, Freud quite often conceptualized things in threes – he even analyzed jokes in a tripartite way, through the relationships of the one making the joke, the object or subject of the joke, and the one who listens to the joke (1905/1976). The tripartite structure can also be referred to as the "topography of the mind," as Freud, ever the doctor, liked to think of psychological structures in a sort of anatomical way.

The three parts of the tripartite structure, as mentioned, are the id, ego, and superego – familiar to those who only colloquially know Freud and those who live and die by his sword. While many know these terms to translate into "instincts," "reality"/"the self," and "morality" (respectively), the definitions are actually quite a bit more nuanced than that. Nancy McWilliams mentions that the translations from Latin are much more appropriate to describe the topography of the mind: the id is "it," the ego is "I," and the superego is "I above" (2004).

The id – "it," if you will – doesn't mean your urges themselves (primarily sex and aggression, the will to love and live or the will to die). It is the drive to *satisfy* those urges; something almost so powerful that it's separate from you, though it informs who you are. To Freud, the id is a representation of your "passions" while the ego is more representative of your "reason and common sense" (Freud, 1989/1923). And the superego, watching over the id's passion and reason-filled domain, is constantly playing a push-and-pull game with the id; it internalizes, negates, reflects and instructs with "its dictatorial 'Thou shalt'" (Freud, 1927). It has two features: the flawless superego, and the punitive ego-ideal that unrealistically strives for perfection. Both portions are derived from a child's earliest object-cathexis, a fancy way of saying one's

DOI: 10.4324/9781003412694-7

emotional attachment to another (usually a primary caregiver). Your caretaker can both do no wrong, as they are a paragon of moral goodness, yet you feel unable to live up to their "ideal" and as one gets older, it takes on a life of its own.

The superego becomes solidified in the mind as a vision of perfection, as it internalizes expectations that it deems valuable, moral, and good. It serves as "the censor" and "the conscience," a version of the ego that rises above the self like a Christ-like vision of purity that one believes they should aspire to (Freud, 1989/1923). And the ego-ideal determines if one's behavior is comparable enough to the superego to feel gratified. More specifically, "this ego-ideal is the precipitate of the old picture of the parents, the expression of admiration for the perfection which the child then attributed to them" (Freud, 1933). Your superego is the textbook, and your ego ideal is the test. And if the ego doesn't pass the exam of acceptable behavior, you subject yourself to guilt, humiliation, and shame. However, from Freud's perspective, guilt was something of a triumph. It meant that your code of ethics was overriding whatever drives you have, creating a sort of superego victory that allows you to feel like whatever you believe a "good person" to be.

Freud used the metaphor that the ego is guiding the id like a rider guides a horse. The horse might sometimes go where it wants to go regardless of the rider's opinion, but the rider is also capable of steering the horse in one direction or another. The superego works to address the id in forceful ways, repressing the Oedipal urges that the id feels so fundamentally intolerable – urges of forbidden, harmful, dangerous, frightening feelings like rage and desire. Like a stern parent, the superego shakes its finger at the id as it screams, flailing its arms and stomping its feet like a child denied ice cream for dinner. "'I did this' is a different experience than 'it came over me'," Jonathan Shedler told McWilliams about the id (2004). And as the id itself is a drive, it compels one to feel or act, pulling them in a direction they didn't intend to go, sometimes to the chagrin of the superego.

The tripartite structure is inherently divided, meaning that the three portions of the self are all psychically divided. In some ways, one could provide the critique that this distances oneself from their desires, almost denying the individual's part in the drama of their indulgences and restrictions. However, to Freud's credit, we all know the feeling of an urge overtaking us, one that we can't control – one that eludes our defenses and pulls us down kicking and screaming. Theorists like Fairbairn and Kohut were more partial to a "unified self" theory that acknowledged the drives as integrated into the ego, a self that was not split off as two seemingly opposing entities (Grotstein, 1980). But alas, they were not yet born to argue their perspectives when this theory was in its infancy.

In the most unembellished of terms, what emerges from this tripartite structure to relate to the world around it is ultimately the ego. The "I" – "ich," to Freud – is the eventual product of this methodology that feels, represses, and interfaces with the world. In German, it is both the self and the functions that make up the self (not just the ego, but the entire tripartite structure and everything that goes with it). Namely, the purpose of this definition is to remember that the ego contains smaller substructures contained therein, and to Beres, "neglecting" this notion "leads to futile semantic conflicts" (1981). It is an individual's version of a supposed "self," the person that you are in response to the emotions and thoughts you have. You take in a stimulus, it brings about feelings in you, you neutralize the darn thing with psychic stomach acid, you spit it out as an identity. A familiar sentiment to the carrot eater (or, rather, to anyone who exists in the world as we know it).

Intrapsychic conflict is when one of the three portions of your tripartite structure contradicts another. If your id, a bastion of aggression, wants to murder your boss, but your superego knows that this would probably have long-standing repercussions, you might find yourself in a bit of an intra-psychic conflict. Intrasystemic conflict, on the other hand, refers to conflicts between the same psychic structure. The most common of these is the id's lust fighting against its hate, but the superego's intrasystemic conflict might include someone who attempts to live up to a lofty paradigm (such as a work ethic, a moral value system, or a standard of emotional regulation) and then punishes themselves when they're unable to succeed in fulfilling it (Lane et al., 1998).

So, we know all about the tripartite structure, the ego, id, and superego, all developing in childhood to create the people we one day become – but how do these structures look in a "normal self" once they've passed through all their various stages and resolved all their Oedipal conflicts (of which we did not cover here, lest this book becomes yet another ode to Freud)?

Kernberg says that one's non-neurotic self "emerges naturally as the tripartite intrapsychic structure is constructed and integrated" (1982). This means that the "self" is integrated and embedded inside the ego, composed of both integrated and unintegrated elements of the tripartite structure. This integration is dependent upon how someone was brought up, how they feel about their primary caregivers, what stages of psychosexual development they might be stuck in, what they might be repressed or defending against, and much, much more. And primarily, repression in particular (though other defenses may also be at play) is the thing that "maintains the dynamic equilibrium of the tripartite structure" in order for the "shadow of unconscious influence and control over the self" to be upheld, even if the unconscious influence is maladaptive or the self-control is but an illusion (Kernberg, 1982). Despite it all, Kernberg continues, these repressed drives "strive for reactivation through invasion of the self's intrapsychic and interpersonal field," meaning that no matter what, even the most integrated of individuals will experience id-driven passions sooner or later (1982).

The tripartite structure lays the basis for every other theory we will be covering in the coming pages. While there's a lot more to it than the brief overview we've just covered, there's yet another reason for a dense foundation of theory covered with such brevity. The knowledge that we have from this section gives us one important lesson: in psychoanalysis, the self attacks, fights, and feels shame about its various parts despite being unified by personhood. Every part of the tripartite structure still exists in one complicated individual who, if you'll forgive the cliché, contains multitudes. The id and superego are almost constantly at odds, with the ego in the middle, just trying to hold it all together. And with this constant inward battle in mind, we can now explore other theoretical perspectives that built off of Freud's ideas to see how that battle looks in one's personality, actions, behaviors, and feelings.

References

Freud, S. (1905/1976). *Jokes and their relation to the unconscious* [New ed.]. London, UK: Penguin.

McWilliams, N. (2004). *Psychoanalytic psychotherapy: A practitioner's guide.* New York: The Guilford Press.

Freud, S. (1989). The ego and the id (1923). *TACD Journal, 17*(1), 5–22. 10.1080/1046171X.1989.12034344

Freud, S. (1933). *New introductory lectures on psychoanalysis.* New York, NY: Norton.

Freud, S. (1927). The ego and the id. The standard edition of the complete psychological works of Sigmund Freud, Volume XIX (1923–1925): The Ego and the Id and Other Works, 1–66.

Grotstein, J.S. (1980). A proposed revision of the psychoanalytic concept of primitive mental states—Part I. Introduction to a newer psychoanalytic metapsychology. *Contemporary Psychoanalysis, 16,* 479–546.

Beres, D. (1981). Self, identity, and narcissism. *Psychoanal Q. Oct, 50*(4), 515–534. PMID: 7302040.

Kernberg, O.F. (1982). Self, ego, affects, and drives. *Journal of the American Psychoanalytic Association, 30*(4), 893–917. 10.1177/000306518203000404

Lane, R. Quintar, B. Goeltz, W.B. (1998). Directions in psychoanalysis. Clinical Psychology Review, 18, 857–88310.1016/s0272-7358(98)00020-8.

Chapter 5

The persona

The tripartite structure has officially been covered in a relative amount of detail. And now, we can move on to other theorists who built upon Freud's ideas, adding their own spices and substituting one ingredient for another. First, we'll cover Carl Jung, who had quite a bit to say about roles and performance in his work. While his theories were only somewhat based upon Freud's classical structure, Jung had a fascination with the self's presentation, how it becomes whole, and how it integrates and distinguishes itself from the noisy outside world. And to make sense of it all, a feature of Jung's theory of how identity is expressed includes something called the persona.

The word *persona*, the cornerstone of his theory on the self, quite literally refers to the masks worn by ancient Greek actors to indicate their characters. The persona exists as something of a compromise between someone and the society they live in – they believe the social environment has certain expectations of them, or they must adhere to certain conventions in order to be treated like one of the in-group. But the persona is tricky, and sometimes, it doesn't seem like a mask – it "feigns individuality, making others and oneself believe that one is individual" (Jung, 1966). And while it is but one part of what Jung considered to be one of the five most prominent features of the "collective unconscious," which are common biological, intellectual, spiritual, and inherited experiences shared unconsciously by humans throughout history, that's a bit beyond our scope today. The alterior side of the persona is the "shadow," including the "anima" and "animus" (among other things) – but for the sake of brevity, we'll simply say that these features of one's personality are generally unconscious and are made known through dreams or fantasies (Friedman, 1966).

The persona develops through an extended and lifelong process in a sort of parallel process to how Jung developed the concept of the persona. While it began as just a way for a child to come into their own away from the mother (1912/1961), it became a much more nuanced idea. Jung never specified about the developmental roots of how the persona is molded, and as a consequence, many theorists believe that it begins when a child enters social settings. This includes family, friends, school, activities, and any other

DOI: 10.4324/9781003412694-8

avenue of communication. When a child's ego is unformed, an individual identifies more with more obvious patterns or ancestral repetitions in the collective unconscious. As a result, their sense of self rests purely in the ideas and notions of what they imagine themselves to be without putting much thought into who they truly are. As the individual grows older, the persona ultimately "consists of the sum of psychic facts that are felt to be personal" as they feel relatable through the ancestral connection one has to the collective unconscious; however, they are "only a mask for the collective psyche" (Jung, 1966). Jung continues that after a while, if one begins to rely on this persona as a means of defining their sense of self, "in an almost magical way the collective psyche begins to determine the individual's fate" (1966). The persona, in a way, can serve as a mechanism to connect one to something beyond themselves. – Stolorow and Atwood refer to this as "pseudo-individuation," as it seems like one is individuation, but they're really just creating a further "vertical split in the psyche" (1977). But when used as a crutch, a persona can become more and more alienated from the inner self as it develops into a forced, kitschy, dramatized performance that one intends to indicate personal depth but just further asserts their need for psychic conformity (Jacobi, 1971).

The way the persona looks is different for everyone, but the following is a solid analogy for the persona of the therapist. Think of a young Aaron Green, Janet Malcolm's subject in *Psychoanalysis: The Impossible Profession,* complementing the lovely tweed jacket of his colleague – one that was almost identical to his own jacket, his favorite jacket to practice therapy in. "I began to look around the institute," he said, "and sure enough, the jacket was all over the place" (1981). Unconsciously for Green, as a starry-eyed psychoanalytic candidate, by sporting the very jacket he saw draped over the bodies of those he aspired to be, he could step into the shoes of the very NYPSI analysts that he idealized so much. For many therapists these days, while the blazer of old has now been shelved, the concept lives on; the popularity of cardigans among therapists has spawned several popular internet memes (@psychotherapymemes, 2020). While these seem like just articles of clothing, they tie into a sort of collective unconscious idea that therapists have regarding who they believe themselves to be – someone who dresses in a certain way, thereby portraying a certain image of themselves.

What one does with the persona is relatively straightforward. Ideally, an individual's true self is realized as they pick apart the persona and really consider from whence it comes. Unconsciously throughout the therapy, aspects of the persona that are "in the way of unconscious integration" and just don't jive with the realized self are thrown right in the psychic garbage. Some say that Jung's own speculations regarding personas were markedly negative, and that he saw them much like Kierkegaard did: one's presentation to the world can end up bogging down one's individuality, and in order to differentiate oneself from others, one must break away from the majority without living in fear of introspection (Kierkegaard, 1967). While the persona is necessary "to make definite impressions upon others," it also assists "to conceal the true nature of the individual" – something of a mediator that "constitutes the compromise between the individual and society" (Hudson, 1978). You see how this could become a problem if impressions meant to conceal turn into impressions manipulated to suppress.

But that's not the whole picture; excess in most any direction can cause things to become destructive, and personas aren't exempt from that scrutiny. Some argue that the persona is a "socially necessary mask" that helps individuals interact with the world in a way that allows them to be socially acceptable without forgoing their individuality (Zinkin, 2008). These theorists believe that once it's been deconstructed and examined rather than relied on out of habit, a persona can be a useful tool to protect the ego. And in the process of questioning and considering one's persona, a period of mourning occurs for the identity one thought they had. Whether it's a compromise formation, or a protective shield, the persona plays a vital role in understanding the ego's relationships with the outside world.

But one thing to remember here (that also applies in other sections, for the record) is something that Jung has in common with Freud – a notable lack of malice. The persona has no marked agenda, just as the superego has no agenda – they are not "good" or "evil." There is no inherent wickedness about these two concepts (though there might be anger or rage attached to them), no ulterior motives to suppress one's personal truths or cramp their style. Any attacks one may internalize from these forces are general indicators of mushy, vulnerable spots in the ego or id, mostly revolving around early childhood relationships with parental figures (Fordham, 1964). Just as well, one should not attempt to live without a persona, lest they become unhinged; Jung, in a somewhat romantic gesture, calls them "hopeless dreamers" destined to be "eternally misunderstood" as they've lost some of the helpful connections you had to the collective unconscious (1966).

To wrap up this small tasting before exploring other theorists, we can use our new knowledge of the persona to begin understanding performance and identity in this context. Personas maintain the balance of one's internal and external states; when one becomes dependent on what they see as externalized social expectations to determine their behavior, thoughts, and feelings, they can lose a sense of who they are beneath the surface. Whether they're infused into one's psyche in early childhood by a parent or crafted by forces of power delineated through functions in society, the mask they form masquerades as identity while it represents an unconscious performance. To Jung, the performance is the false expression of identity, and the identity is the thing hidden beneath the persona. Ultimately, the goal of acknowledging the persona to Jung is to recognize and live alongside the persona using *individuation*; breaking away from what you believe others expect of you to become an individual. By allowing one's persona to become a realistic mirror of your true self, one can integrate their personality into their perception of a collective psychic position. The performance then becomes a way to relate to the world rather than a way to hide yourself from it. And Jung isn't the only one who thought along those lines.

References

Jung. (1966). In G. Adler & R.F.C. Hull (Eds.), *Collected works of C.G. Jung. vol. 7, two essays in analytical psychology*. Princeton, NJ: Princeton University Press. Republished in 1967.

Jung, C.G., & Hull, R.F.C. (1912/1961). *Jung contra Freud: The 1912 New York lectures on the theory of psychoanalysis* (REV-Revised). Princeton University Press. http://www.jstor.org/stable/j.ctt7s8mf

Atwood, G.E., & Stolorow, R.D. (1977). Metapsychology, reification and the representational world of C. G. Jung. *International Review of Psychoanalysis, 4,* 197–213.

Jacobi, J. (1971). Die Seelenmaske. Olten, Walter Verlag (trans. E. Begg as Masks of the soul, London, Darton, Longman and Todd, 1976).

Malcolm, J. (1981). *Psychoanalysis the impossible profession* (1st ed.). Knopf. Retrieved December 14 2022 from http://catalog.hathitrust.org/api/volumes/oclc/7575595.html.

@psychotherapymemes. (2020, July 27). Nobody: Therapists: Hm which of my 18 cardigans shall I wear today? [Tweet]. Retrieved from https://twitter.com/psychotherapym8/status/1287782439046148096

Kierkegaard, S. (1967/1996). *Papers and journals* (A. Hannay Trans.). London, UK: Penguin Books. Republished on 1996.

Hudson, W.C. (1978). Persona and defence mechanisms. *Journal of Analytical Psychology, 23,* 54–62.

Zinkin, L. (2008). Your self: Did you find it or did you make it?. *Journal of Analytical Psychology, 53,* 389–406.

Fordham, F. (1964). The care of regressed patients and the child archetype. *Journal of Analytical Psychology, 9,* 61–73.

Friedman, M. (1966). Jung's Image of Psychological Man. Psychoanalytic Review. 53D, 4: 95–108.

Chapter 6

The False Self and the idealized image

Here we have a delicious course with two tasty treats for the price of one: child psychologist D.W. Winnicott, and adult psychologist Karen Horney. Many draw parallels between Jung's theory of the persona and Winnicott's musings on identity. And even Horney's theories likewise have loose echoes of the persona present (much to the chagrin of all those who believe Jung was nothing more than a quixotic philosopher), as they both speak of some sort of unattainable standard one sets for the presentation of their identities. As we've mentioned, you'll start to see a pattern: fundamentally, this is about who we are through what we portray, and if what we express matches or contradicts what we feel. *Alors, mangeons!*

The False Self

Winnicott's True and False Self theory operates in a way that some would consider an elaboration on the persona; though they came from distinctively varied places in terms of the developmental and theoretical nature of their arguments, there's no doubt that the two theories are adjacent. Throughout his extensive career, one of Winnicott's leitmotifs was how individuals cultivate an inner life and construct fantasies in their own personal realities. His focus was often on personal meaning, which is determined by this secret, vivid inner life. And often, he saw patients who were cruising through life on autopilot, living in a world that wasn't their own; namely, patients who performed their way through life without a face under the mask. With no creativity, no fantasies, these patients felt they were constantly adjusting to the world around them, which Winnicott says goes back to childhood.

In Winnicottian theory, raising an infant isn't just about fulfilling their basic needs and calling it a day (1953). An infant's mind is like a series of wish-driven vignettes – "*I'm hungry!*" or "*I'm tired!*" or "*I'm lonely!*" – but they're not quite an integrated self, as they're still acclimating to the concept of being alive. And in his theory, the first few moments of the baby's life include a primary caregiver who is (or rather, should be) entirely focused on the needs of the baby, such as feeding it, putting it to bed, and snuggling with it.

DOI: 10.4324/9781003412694-9

The baby's first year of life, they've got it made; every time they're hungry, food appears, and every time they're tired, a bed appears. This gives an infant what Winnicott calls *subjective omnipotence*, or the feeling that the child, a god of their own world, can create and destroy things on demand in accordance with their need of the hour.

However, as the child gets older, the primary caregiver begins going back to a life of their own. And as the baby realizes that their needs aren't going to be met instantaneously anymore, they develop a sense of *objective reality*. This is the dreaded notion that other people in the world exist, and life is full of external stimuli. Regretfully for this infant, sometimes, you've got to accommodate their needs as well as your own. As the infant learns this, they begin to bring together parts of themselves that feel like they have control over their environment and parts that don't. And with solid caregiving, these two experiences can live side by side.

Ultimately, a fully formed ego has both *subjective omnipotence,* which allows one to be the god of their own wishes and fantasies, and *objective reality*, which shows that you're sometimes dependent on others (Winnicott, 1953). Living with these two phenomena turns a well-adjusted baby into a well-adjusted adult. They become someone who relates to the world internally and externally, both maintaining core parts of themselves and adjusting situationally to accommodate their environments. And if the primary caregiver's parenting is a bit lackluster, the infant's psychological development is frozen in time. The rest of their personalities grow around this intrapsychic life suspended in animation. And hence, the True and False Selves are born.

The False Self, much like the persona, "describes the adaptation that the subject has to make in order to live within his social context" as it becomes a "vigilant caretaker" of the True Self (Skelton, 2006). This True Self, a place of genuine desire, is this undeveloped core around which the False Self is constructed. The experience of a False Self is almost like living in Winnicott's *objective reality* and keeping oneself constantly affixed on external stimuli. But just like the persona, the True and False Selves don't represent the untruthful person you're pretending to be and the truly authentic person deep down inside. The False Self's varying degrees are "ranging from the healthy, polite aspect of the self to the truly split-off compliant False Self," and in the worst-case scenario "a child grows up to be an actor" (Winnicott & Khan, 1958; Winnicott, 1965). Winnicott's view of the self is about assimilation and ego protection; the False Self must be assessed. Some theorists say that many modern patients feel like Winnicott's archetype – someone floating through life unable to access the authenticity of their True Self as it remains hidden deep inside of a False Self that they cannot break through (Bader, 1995).

Though the False Self is performance, it combines with the True Self to create identity. Without a False Self, the yolk and whites of one's egg are boiled without a shell, the contents losing their shape, splitting apart, whipping wildly hither and yon in the turbulent water of reality. This extremely thrilling inner life, the True Self, is meant for you and only you. It is a realm over which you have complete control, as the *subjective omnipotence* you cultivated early in life is the "healthy foundation from which the self develops" (Davies, 2009). But it's got to stay concealed. Otherwise, an overwhelming sense of *subjective omnipotence* can turn into delusions of grandeur or magical thinking. In your own mind, you are the architect of your entire world. And if that grandiosity is taken and used as a tool by the False Self, it transforms from something internally known to something externally performed – "I am a model of kindness," or "compliancy," "the model student," or "the model child, as I have control over how everyone sees me." And in this Winnicottian conceptualization of identity, that's where identity is lost to performance: when one believes they can control how others see them.

The idealized image

Moving right along. In Jung's theory, one must integrate a persona into their sense of self – one's internal preoccupation with an external presentation) needs to be reconciled. And Winnicott's theory is more centered on highlighting the True Self while the False Self learns to adapt around it. But to one theorist, these somewhat performative facades aren't at all beneficial to integrate into one's whole self, even if one is under the impression that it's an important part of your personality. Psychoanalyst and proto-feminist Karen Horney gives us an example of such unproductive external influences dominating one's sense of themselves in the form of the real self and the idealized image. And much like the warnings present at the beginning of each section, Horney-lovers beware; this crash course glazes over many a gory detail.

Horney's child is one that was born with the urge to self-actualize and is always going towards a life that cultivates meaningful values, goals, and relationships. However, this child's development can be impeded in a number of ways by their primary caregivers. To Horney, a child's self-actualization is put on the backburner when people in their environment are too "wrapped up in their neuroses to be able to love the child" (1950). As a response to this lack of love, the child doesn't develop a sense of belonging, resulting in an all-consuming *basic anxiety* that permeates their every action. To cope with this basic anxiety, they relate to people in three ways: *moving towards* (becoming needy), *moving away from* (becoming isolated), or *moving against* (becoming angry and lashing out). At the root of it all, though the child has something within them that wants to become, that wants to evolve – a "central inner force, common to all human beings and yet unique in each, which is the deep source of growth" (1950). This can be called the *real self.*

These three "moving" coping mechanisms evolve throughout life, but ultimately, the more someone orients their lives around dealing with basic anxiety, the less they feel equipped to handle everyday life. Their lives are then structured around avoiding these negative feelings, and to do so, they make a sort of internal compromise. A child's inner self and their fundamental needs go to the backburner as their only focus in life is on maintaining a feeling of safety. In a way, they're no longer in control of the metaphorical vehicle, and instead, the person in charge is one they've constructed to defend against hurt, pain, and misunderstanding.

Now that the idealized image is in the driver's seat, creating a version of the child the world comes to know the child to be, it eventually becomes more real than the real self, as it fulfills all the child's needs – the need to be safe, the need to avoid danger, the need to have their fantasies fulfilled by imagination. As the child's idealized image solidifies into an adult, character constellations are compulsively and neurotically formed. The curation of one's identity becomes about doing whatever possible to avoid situations in which the ego is harmed, and the idealized image is now a version of the individual that has control over their environment in a way that the vulnerable ego does not.

Unfortunately, this formation can be damaging not just for the ego, but for one's relationship with others – the desperate attempt to maintain this idealized image results in behaviors that could be considered harmful neurotic pride, a defense against insecurity, feeling unworthy, or feeling perpetuates toxic, unhelpful undercurrents in one's inner life. The neurotic pride makes someone "alienated" from themselves, "divided," and "lifting himself in his mind above the crude reality of himself and others" (Horney, 1950). This contrasts with the real self, who has the characteristics most authentic to the patient's true wants, needs, and internal compass. Falling prey to this dynamic renders the idealized self adored, and the real self ignored; "the central inner conflict is one between the constructive forces of the real self and the obstructive forces of the pride system," between growth in a thoughtful, healthy way that nurtures the real self, "and the drive to prove in actuality the perfection of the idealized self" (Horney, 1950).

While this might seem like predominantly internal notions that roll around in an individual's head without really making contact with the outside world, the patient's idealized self emerges in their actions in unconscious and unfortunate ways. In particular, the idealized self presents "the tendency to experience internal processes as if they occurred outside oneself"; one then regards "external factors [as] responsible for one's difficulties" (Horney, 1945). She compares this to the adjacent Jungian concept of extraversion, where "the most frequent and essential decisions and actions are determined, not by subjective values but by objective relations" (Jung, 1923). This can manifest as one's inclinations to rely on others to reassure them that this construction of who they wish to be is legitimately themselves.

One might remember Winnicott's False Self being used to exert a measure of control over the way one is perceived, and the idealized image functions in the same way. As we circle back to performance in identity, we find the idealized image showing up to our dinner party in furs and diamond jewelry.

If the False Self is sincere, the idealized image is the sincerest; if the False Self is kind, the idealized image is the kindest; and if the False Self is perfect, well, you get the picture. To Horney, one's entire internal process is fixated on defending the performance they see to be their identity, and beneath it all there may very well be nothing of substance. If there's nothing beneath the performance, one would assume that it simply becomes the identity, as nowhere in our cookbook does it say that identity must be authentic or inauthentic. But it remains to be seen if anyone would be content living life that way in the long term.

And wouldn't you know it, what timing! Our guest of honor has just walked in, and we're onto our next course; we've melded identity and performance art, we have a sense of how they fit together. And now, we're ready to explore how it all fits into the larger context of the therapist's performance and the performance therapist themselves.

References

Winnicott, D.W. (1953). Transitional objects and transitional phenomena – A study of the first not-me possession. *International Journal of Psycho-Analysis, 34*, 89–97.

Skelton. (2006). *The Edinburgh international encyclopedia of psychoanalysis Edinburgh.* Edinburgh, Scotland: Edinburgh University Press. Web.

Winnicott, & Khan, M.M.R. (1958). *Through paediatrics to psycho-analysis* (1st ed.). England: Routledge. 10.4324/9780429484001. Web.

Winnicott. (1965). *The maturational processes and the facilitating environment: Studies in the theory of emotional development.* England: Haithi Trust. Web.

Bader, M.J. (1995). Authenticity and the psychology of choice in the analyst. *Psychoanalytic Quarterly, 64*, 282–305.

Davies, J.E. (2009). Considering "Self-Ful" desire. *Psychoanalytic Psychology, 26*, 310–321.

Horney. (1950). *Neurosis and human growth: The struggle toward self-realization.* New York: W. W. Norton. Web.

Horney. (1945). *Our inner conflicts: A constructive theory of neurosis.* New York: W.W. Norton. Republished on 1966.

Jung. (1923/1971/2016). *Psychological types* (H. G. Baynes Trans.). Eastford, CT: Martino Fine Books. Print.

Part III

Performance (of the therapist)

Our education in performance art and psychoanalytic conceptualizations of identity is complete – give yourself a round of applause for making it through. And now, we move on to performance, the old can of worms; the "false," maybe even the fake (or so it is often conceived). On one hand, we have performance within the concept of selfhood that we were just exploring. It's the thing you show to the world as a means of protecting whatever's beneath. Performance can be anything from a banal work ego to a crispy, glazed façade of defenses formed in fear, concealing the vulnerable, tantalizing jelly filling of the true self inside. On the other hand, we have performance through performance art. Ball, Tzara, and their comrades Yoko Ono or Emilia Fart declared their most inner selves to the world dressed in feather boas, howling in an untranslatable conniption, finding vulnerability and truth in nonsense and insanity. Which one is the performance?

With our recent review, we have the building blocks necessary to begin understanding how we can transpose the former's view of performance onto the latter. Expressions and feelings about identity in performance art are inner truths (True Selves, real selves, and the like) spoken using False Selves and personas. The performance artist engages in pleasure in its most intense form: turning body, appearance, and action – one's entire existence – into an abstract, intangible, emotion-laden testimonial. They take the idealized self and hold it up as a paragon of expression while simultaneously critiquing and parodying it. It is the id, and it is the superego – it is the chaos and the presence of mind to regulate its communication. And with this mindset, we can shift our focus to what might be the most important course so far: *performance* – of the therapist, that is.

"Performance" – A dirty word?

Like an opera singer belting a song in a language they do not know, the performer can be seen as someone who is mimicking an act rather than speaking from a place of innermost personal knowledge. This is especially

DOI: 10.4324/9781003412694-10

the case when a therapist is considered to be conducting a performance, as it denotes a certain type of hollow imitation of empathy and connection. It might even seem like an attack against one's person to hear that they could perform in the room, as to many, it contradicts with a sense of intimacy, authenticity, and transparency. To the untrained eye, performance and performativity are the same, with some underlying current of deceptiveness or bravado layered in the act. And the performer, one who is attempting to imitate something that they're not, becomes someone who pretends rather than someone who is, as if the two concepts are mutually exclusive.

However, if there's anything we've learned from our explorations into identity, a performance can be as real or unreal as the individual executing that performance. One's intentional attempt at portraying something (a character, an idea, an emotion) doesn't mean that these performances are "faked," that they're inauthentic or artificial. Their depth may not be in the act itself, but in the reasons why the act is performed. How performance looks, whether the act is convincing or unconvincing, believable or unbelievable, isn't necessarily the main feature – though it certainly isn't immaterial, as it can serve as a healthy barometer for how in tune one is with their inner needs. The inner needs, though, are the most important feature of this equation, for without a glut of (sometimes quite hidden) content beneath the surface, no performance can be conducted in the first place. And sometimes, these slips are unconscious, as the False self, the idealized image, and the persona can sneak out to protect the ego when the individual doesn't even realize it needs protecting. Performance is not a dirty word. It is a necessary one. Because without it, one cannot communicate with their external worlds in a way that also preserves the integrity of their identities.

The brutal truth of individual identity is the core of performance art, just as it is with psychoanalysis. And these two domains are so marked by uncontrollable drives, by deep and unwieldy vigor, they can dominate and sway spaces, leaving collateral damage in their wake. In that case, how can either of these things be constructed? Held or bound by parameters? And how, then, can we begin to think about the therapist – whose mark of individuality must inherently be *contained* by structure? While each patient requires varied interventions for successful treatment, in the most traditional of psychoanalytic viewpoints, the therapist exists only to reflect the worldview of the patient they are seeing at the moment and not to let their distinctiveness run wild. It seems almost counterintuitive to integrate the performance artist and therapist in this way – the latter necessitates control while the former denounces it. But remember that the performance artist does outline how their performance will work. They must buy the Volkswagen they want to crucify themselves atop or find the perfect tree to climb up in the nude. The performance artist needs a frame of their own making to tear down the composition of the art world, facilitating deeper understanding about the human condition. And the therapist needs a frame to tear down the composition of the patient's defenses, to facilitate deeper understanding about the human condition as well.

Fundamentally, these forces mirror each other in the most basic of ways. Think of the tenants of dadaism: anti-art is made with humor and autonomy, with whimsy and emotion, with natural off-the-cuff flow and irrational confusion. Do these descriptors sound familiar? Do they paint the picture of the ideal therapeutic experience one so desperately aims to achieve – something so human, and yet so inexplicably surreal? While the "rules" in therapy might seem different, the end goal is the same: understanding humanity in ways we cannot truly put to paper. And the format? The inception of psychoanalysis drew from an inability to use the then common terminology to discuss the brains of patients in a helpful yet scientific way. A dissatisfaction in the way things were previously done. The abject need to create their own language, exhausted with the pre-existing, ineffectual theory, the "words that other people have invented" (Ball & Pinoncelli, 1916). And from this came not only the persona of The Ideal Therapist, but his many beloved children, unique in their own ways, yearning for that same kind of exploration and adventure, fueled by enterprise and ingenuity. Sometimes in ways that reflect the direction of the field at large, and sometimes in ways that reflect their own cocktail of analytic and philosophical interests.

Bon appetite!

Unfortunately for the therapist (who I'm sure would have a much easier job if people were simple) individuality is an absolutely necessary function of each and every person on earth. No matter how much one has been trained to maintain self-restraint, they always have been and always will be themselves, and no one else – though even what "being themselves" means is different for everyone. It has been said that the goal of the therapist is to "leave themselves at the door", so to speak, and that concept is the backbone of many an analytic theory. However, there is an express reason that theory and practice are spoken of in two realms, and while the ideal is to integrate them, it's a long and winding road to get there; uphill both ways, frankly, as one is always battling against unveiling their own individuality.

So, how does one assert the individuality of a performance artist while also securing themselves in a steady state of identification with The Therapist, this abstract imago outside themselves? Is there a key to unlocking individuality in the therapeutic relationship that we have not yet addressed, one that can answer this question?

Perhaps so, as our guest has made his introductions and is seated at the table. He is the archetype for how the therapist performs using tenants of performance art. He is ready to be picked apart and chewed on. He will give us a recipe to take home and try in our own kitchens: one part *structural performance,* one part *emotional performance,* and one part *patient.* And he goes by the name of the *performance therapist.*

Reference

Ball, H., & Pinoncelli, P. (Eds.). (1916). *Le manifeste dada (the dada manifesto).* Saint-Étienne, France: Le Réalgar. Web.

Chapter 7

The structural performance

Now we have the task of understanding the first ingredient of the performance therapist: the structural performance. But first, we should clarify something. The main reason that we break down the therapist's performance into these two categories of structure and emotion is because performance art can be thought of comparably. Though performance art is rarely broken down into those terms, it can be conceptualized like this: many performance artists have a background in either other types of art or the general subject they're performing about. Casey Jenkins could not perform *Casting off My Womb* did she not know how to knit (2013), and even Bettina Behjat Banayan graduated from the French Culinary Institute before frosting a cake on a New York City subway (2014). While a performance artist doesn't necessarily need to have professional training in order to take on performance art as their own, they need to have a frame they tap into in order to display pieces in all their glory. Their structure provides the setting, tools, time, and place – the time slot you paid for in the Museum of Modern Art, the credit card you used to buy a microphone, the outfit you picked out just for the occasion. And when they structure is in place, you can unleash the emotional performance, screaming noise poems to the masses (Ono, 2010). But we'll get to that part later.

Onto the structural performance. Most simply, this performance is one that integrates knowledge from *education*, *practical*, and *clerical* items with the perspective from which you approach the treatment. In simpler terms, it is the nuts and bolts of your practice, the foundational egg whites of the psychological soufflé that your patients will consume. As for why a therapist's structural performance relates to performance art, the answer is simple: the therapist ingests the carrots of their own practical experience, digests them, and displays them in a way all their own.

One's structural performance is defined by a few key things: who you read, what supervisors you have, what school you go to, and what theories you identify with most. Additionally, the structural performance also includes the frame; the timing of sessions, such as how long your days are, how many minutes you allow a session to go on, and even how you handle running late. Then there's scheduling – how you communicate with your patient about a

DOI: 10.4324/9781003412694-11

reschedule, or how you handle when they ask for a different time. There are also vacations, namely how a patient is notified of a vacation or how it's treated in the session. Even the manner in which one gets patients, perhaps through a program like Headspace or Alma, is considered in the frame. These are the bricks with which your practice is built, as it includes how it grows, progresses, and maintains.

The structural performance in some ways can seem pretty cut and dry, as one's educational history, electronic medical record (EMR) software, and books in their library are all measurable. But everyone's experience is different, as is everyone's theoretical orientation. It's all what Bernstein calls "a matter of taste;" a rather Marinetti-like comparison (2001). Therapists have the freedom to choose which theory they follow, how they get their patients, how they communicate with their patients outside of sessions, and how they monitor their patients' progress. Every soufflé is different, as is every practice, but the structure must be there all the same lest your whole practice deflates.

Here, we'll be focusing mostly on the latter portion of the structural performance definition: the treatment perspective. This is the knowledge base that the therapist has received over years of training that helps them create a style substantiated by certain technical texts. Each type of therapy, of which at this point there are many, has its own different style of "performance"; this is to say, their own version of how to act in the room, and what to say. There's not necessarily an instruction packet filled with exact phrases and responses. But in Freud's words, psychoanalysis is a game of chess; the beginning and end are somewhat guided, but the intermediate segments are highly varied; they depend on the patient, the therapist, and everything in between (Fenichel, 1939). One's perspective can be informed by analytic or psychodynamic literature, cognitive behavioral therapy (CBT), dialectical behavioral therapy (DBT), and more – sometimes, even a hodge-podge of everything. This perspective can also be attained through schooling, such as an advanced degree, through education from supervisors or mentors, and sometimes even in continuing education programs. But no matter what, this type of knowledge is a necessity for the therapist to have, and one's structural performance is just as important as any other feature of their practice. Without this sort of training, a therapist is no longer a therapist, but a friend, mentor, advisor, or life coach – just like a soufflé without eggs is simply a béchamel sauce.

Why exactly is this a performance in the way that performance art is a performance? Because what's learned in training may, in fact, be counter-intuitive to how a person might act if they were driven by impulse – though at times, the impulse or inner voice drives the work. It is channeled and ex-pressed desires existing only in the feedback loop of your experience and practice. It is unscripted, moment-to-moment, and never ending – the act stays with you long after you leave the session, and feeds into the entire image one has of themselves as a therapist. But at the same time, it is planned, crafted, and well thought-out. The structural performance isn't just about executing techniques that one reads in a textbook with precision and grace. In totality, the voices of their teachers are then integrated into their own voice, inverting, subverting, and rethinking systems they once knew. It is not about performing the structure exactly as you learned it. It is about performing the structure as you eventually come to know it.

And there we have the structural performance; you know how to act, as you've been taught, told, educated, or shown with experience. In this way, the therapist is embodying the very structure of their practice into the way they act and how they relate to the world around them when they're in the metaphorical blazer (or cardigan). It is taught in roleplays, in transcriptions, in the taping and reviewing of sessions, in the classroom, and in the supervision room. And it is executed like this.

How does a structurally psychoanalytic performance look?

While structural performances come in all shapes and sizes, here, we'll be talking about the *psychoanalytic structural performance* that embraces a therapist's partially (or fully) psychoanalytic or psychodynamic background. One certainly doesn't need to be a purist in order to practice in this way, as many therapists take bits and pieces from analysis and pepper them into their own technique. And, as always, this is but an example – facets of any thera-peutic modality can be inserted into this model to break down the various learned ways in which a therapist might act with a patient. Each type of therapy has principles describing attitudes, actions, or responses that a ther-apist should have.

All of the following technical points outlined by Freud himself are what one could call the basic format of a structurally psychoanalytic performance. As some of these responses and actions are not necessarily the first inclination of many in an informal dialogue with friends, family, or peers, one must first learn how and why certain statements might be therapeutic or untherapeutic in nature. While this process might begin as a conscious parroting of one's instructors, eventually, one hopes to have a seamless integration of method-ology into one's therapeutic identity. The main points explored below are the most obvious, and the most prolific in classically analytic practices: *evenly suspended attention,* the rules of *abstinence* and *neutrality,* and in the context of all that, *rapport.*

Evenly suspended attention, the first of these directives addressed, "consists simply in not directing one's notice to anything in particular"; if not, "one point will be fixed in his mind with particular clearness and some other will be correspondingly disregarded," leading to a particular issue "following [the therapist's] expectations or inclinations" (Freud, 1912). This, in more basic terms, means that a therapist should not instruct the patient, directly or indirectly, to hyper-focus on certain details of the case that might dissuade them from free associating. If evenly suspended attention is deployed outside of the analytic situation, the other party may respond with limited enthusiasm. But in session, it is necessary to remember that all information given by the patient is pertinent, and no road should be closed off in the map of their minds.

More often than not, the therapist must make a conscious decision to engage in this reaction, hence, a technique of performance. Maintaining evenly suspended attention isn't second nature to most for a number of reasons. Primarily, facilitating an environment of free association isn't necessary that common in daily conversation, as two parties hopping from one point to another can result in simultaneous monologuing, like two toddlers in a playpen. And usually, certain topics are off-limits due to social stigma or mindfulness about etiquette, turning free association into a bit of a faux pas. Holding a frame that shies away from the more unsavory id-driven topics in life is but a human impulse – avoiding topics that one's evenly-suspended attention, ideally, doesn't find too unsavory.

Abstinence, the next classical technique, ensures "that the patient's suffering, to a degree that is in some way or other effective, does not come to an end prematurely" (Freud, 1919). The therapist is attempting to *abstain* from any sort of personal investment in the patient by means of gratifying needs through judgments, personal admissions, praises and affirmations, or anything that eliminates their impartiality. While an analytic technique like evenly suspended attention maintains the therapist must not focus too much on any one subject, abstinence asserts that the analyst must not shy away from patient's emotions that are difficult to process. And paired with abstinence we have *neutrality*, which encompasses the notion that the therapist chooses not to impose themselves on the patient in any way. In Janet Malcolm's words, these techniques means that the therapist is:

> mild, colorless, self-effacing, uninterfering, and undemanding as he is able to make it, and as it is toward no one else in his life - with the paradoxical (and now absolutely predictable) result that the patient reacts with stronger, more vivid and intense personal feelings to his bland shadowy figure than he does more to the clearly delineated and provocative figures in his life.
>
> (Malcolm, 1981)

The reason that abstinence can be considered a feature of the performance is that it may, for some, operate in contrast with the urge to console (or at least de-escalate) when one sees another in distress. In the same article, Freud mentions that the therapist should not try to manage or control the patient's distress, and in fact, their "need and longing should be allowed to persist" in the transference "in order that they may serve as forces impelling [the patient] to do work and to make changes" (1919). The same can be said not only for longing but also for feelings of anger, resentment, sadness, or misunderstanding. To indulge these feelings would be putting a Band-Aid on an open wound, in the paraphrased words of Freud, and while it's important for the therapist to inwardly maintain empathy, outwardly they must embody nothing but a willingness to explore emotions the patient may find it hard to sit with.

Rapport, the final example to touch on, is "to attach … the person [to] the doctor. To ensure this, nothing need be done but to give him time" (Freud, 1913). Freud mentions that the patient may immediately attach to the therapist through transference, and that "if from the start one takes up any standpoint other than one of sympathetic understanding, such as a moralizing one", that initial projection can easily be shattered (1913). Building rapport through our old friend neutrality rather than sympathy can feel unnatural, but Freud argues that one does not necessarily need to be overtly affirming in order to build a bond of trust. The neutrality, if correctly implemented, is its own form of empathy; it takes shape as the patient begins to feel reassured that they're simply being listened to.

With such rules for how to behave, rules present in any modality of therapy (even if the rules are "there are no rules"), we begin to realize how easy it is for a therapist to slip into identifying with a persona. One who embodies each one of these facets and more becomes a sort of definitive Analyst, one that some therapists (particularly psychodynamic ones) end up seeing as the archetype from which they should either adhere or rebel. He is capable of being a perfect space to reflect "the patient's unconscious phantasies of his parental images, or parts of them", and if this relationship is maintained with strength and intention, these will "come fully into play, manifesting themselves by means of transference to the analyst" (Foulkes, 1965). Freud analogously compared the psychoanalyst to a surgeon, one "who puts aside all of his own feelings, including that of human sympathy, and concentrates his mind on one single purpose, that of performing the operation as skillfully as possible" (Gelso & Kanninen, 2017). Ironically, Marinetti would say that a declaimer is someone who's inclined to "dress anonymously, "dehumanize his voice," "dehumanize his face," and simultaneously "be a tireless creator and inventor" – a definition that Freud may indeed find relatable (1916). But how realistic is a performance this rigid? And do all structural performances have to translate verbatim from theory to practice?

How theory becomes personal: Performance to technique

Only from this distinct Freudian basis of the measured analyst can we begin to formulate our further argument of going beyond *acting like* a therapist to attentively *performing* as a therapist like any Marina Abromovic or Hugo Ball. Any actor can study a role, and whether they buy into the character or not, they can recite the lines – sometimes with a fascinating level of feeling that entices and enraptures the audience. But the therapist was never meant to entice or enrapture. He was simply meant to be, as any living human is. To Freud's metaphor once again, a surgeon is not *acting* a surgery, he *performs* a surgery, as he *is* a surgeon. And what is a surgeon but a human, studied and experienced, in a doctor's coat – one that frames their humanity without attempting to stifle it?

To many, the orthodox Freudian definition of how a therapist performs feels a bit outdated or stiff. And Freud's adherence to unemotional inquiry to maintain the integrity of the analytic technique is striking – "I sit by a sickbed in order to observe", Freud tells his wife in a letter, "I treat human suffering as an object ... it can't be done any other way" (Gay, 1988). And in this particular structural performance, a therapist can seem "distant, aloof, and without feelings for the patient" (Eagle, 2011). Even the most experienced therapist knows that while these tenets are helpful to maintain a psychodynamic frame, leaning too hard into any modality can result in creating a sort of silo mentality in which potentially beneficial or useful insights are blocked off by one's inability to think outside the epistemological box. In fact, Fairbairn notes that adhering to a sort of rigid technique of analysis "is liable to defensive exploitation, however unconscious this may be, in the interests of the analyst and at the expense of the patient" (1958).

This critique of a psychoanalytic performance – that leaning too much on structure can be a problem in practice – is but one of many criticisms on our buffet. Stifling the humanity therapists attempt to frame with structure is quite the undertaking, and though a therapist may study, rehearse, and rehash, their ultimate goal is integration rather than assimilation (Hallgrímsson, 1994). An oddly commonplace issue in modernity is the assumption that an excess of any structure will fill all gaps in one's practice. And if this studious act is performed well enough, a convincingly "good therapist" will begin to emerge. This is evidenced in the sheer number of weekend courses, workshops, and seminars, some available at discounted rates if you buy in bulk[1]. Acceptance and Commitment Therapy (ACT), Eye Movement Desensitization and Reprocessing Therapy (EMDR), Accelerated Resolution Therapy (ART), and other "numerous specialty certifications are awarded on this basis of existing accomplishments [holding a degree/licensure] and attendance at a single educational workshop" (Rosen et al., 2020). In some ways, one has a readymade identity based upon structure alone. But as Rosen finds, if an eighth grader with no psychoeducation can pass the final exam of a $199 weekend seminar to become a Certified Clinical Trauma Professional, maybe there's more to therapeutic identity than just the letters after one's name (Rosen et al. 2020). A single-mindedness about maintaining the façade of learnedness can slowly transform from an eager practitioner to an idealized image, convincing themselves that quantity is the equivalent of quality – as even the most sumptuous looking of apples can be made of wax.

"I think therapists are interested in helping as best as they can," says social worker Jason Peng (personal communication, 2022). He continues, and yes, that includes more short-term approaches – EMDR, solutions-focused, CBT, MI. The field is infatuated with the rate of recovery. So we search for the next best thing, wanting that illusion [of results]. And as long as there is a market, then there will be sellers who come around and promise it.

Just as one differentiates themselves and their therapeutic identity by using various theories piecemeal in accordance with different patients, one must not assume that the entire argument of the performance therapist rests only on the structural performance. A writer learns the rules of grammar front to back, only to become e.e. cummings; a painter goes to years of technically precise art school only to become Picasso. Strupp even goes so far as to call theoretical orientation "an overrated variable;" "in the end," he says, "each therapist develops his or her own style and the 'theoretical orientation' fades into the background" (1978). And a therapist munches on the carrots of classical Freudian techniques, or Lacanian, Kleinian, Fairbairnian ones, from EFT to EMDR or any other acronym under the sun, just to become their own special shade of performer, from a burnt umber to a neon orange. Even if one amalgamates as much knowledge as they possible can, they're still digesting it and interpreting it through their own palates – "wherever you learn, there you are," or something like that. And wherever the structural performance goes, the *emotional performance* is sure to follow.

Note

1   ProfessionalPsychSeminars.com, a Continued Education (CE) service, offers 10% off if you buy two or more classes. The Knowledge Tree, another CE service, offers 20% off a purchase of five classes or more. I could go on, but I'd rather give free publicity if I knew I was getting something good out of the deal.

References

Jenkins, C. (2013). *Casting off my womb*. [Performance]. Darwin City, Australia: Darwin Visual Arts Association.
Banayan, B.B. (2014). *Subway cake performance*. [Performance]. New York.
Ono, Y. (2010). *Voice piece for soprano & wish tree.*[Performance]. New York: Museum of Modern Art.
Bernstein, A. (2001). Psychotherapy as a performing art: The role of therapeutic style. *Modern Psychoanalysis*, *26*, 183–190.
Fenichel, O. (1939). Problems of psychoanalytic technique. *The Psychoanalytic Quarterly*, *8*(1), 57–87. 10.1080/21674086.1939.11925377
Rosen, G.M., Washburn, J.J., & Lilienfeld, S.O. (2020). Specialty certifications for mental health practitioners: A cautionary case study. *Professional Psychology: Research and Practice*, *51*(6), 545–549. 10.1037/pro0000324

Freud, S. (1912). Recommendations to physicians practising psycho-analysis. In Strachey, J., Freud, A., Strachey, A. & Tyson, A. (Eds.), *The standard edition of the complete psychological works of Sigmund Freud Volume XII (1911–1913): The Case of Schreber, Papers on Technique and Other Works* (pp. 109–120). London, England: Hogarth Press.

Freud, S. (1919). Lines of advance in psycho-analytic therapy. In Strachey, J., Freud, A., Strachey, A. & Tyson, A. (Eds.), *The standard edition of the complete psychological works of Sigmund Freud, Volume XVII: An Infantile Neurosis and Other Works* (pp. 157–168). London, England: Hogarth Press.

Malcolm, J. (1981). *Psychoanalysis the impossible profession* (1st ed.). New York: W.W. Norton.

Freud, S. (1913). On beginning the treatment (further recommendations on the technique of psycho-analysis I). In Strachey, J., Freud, A., Strachey, A. & Tyson, A. (Eds.), *The standard edition of the complete psychological works of Sigmund Freud, Volume XII: The Case of Schreber, Papers on Technique and Other Works* (pp. 121–144). London, England: Hogarth Press.

Foulkes, D. (1965). *Therapeutic group analysis* (American ed.). New York: International Universities Press.

Gelso, C.J., & Kanninen, K.M. (2017). Neutrality revisited: On the value of being neutral within an empathic atmosphere. *Journal of Psychotherapy Integration, 27*(3), 330–341. 10.1037/int0000072

Marinetti, F.T. Ed., & Rainey, L. (1916/2009). *Dynamic and synoptic declamation.* Futurism: an anthology. New Haven, CT: Yale University Press.

Eagle. (2011). *From classical to contemporary psychoanalysis: A critique and integration.* New York: Taylor and Francis. Web.

Fairbairn, W.D. (1958). On the nature and aims of psycho-analytical treatment. *International Journal of Psychoanalysis, 39,* 374–385.

Gay, P. (1988). *Freud: A life for our time.* New York: W. W. Norton.

Hallgrímsson, Ó. (1994) "Forgotten" theory. *Journal of Clinical Psychoanalysis, 3,* 407–428.

Strupp, H.H. (1978). The therapist's theoretical orientation: An overrated variable. *Psychotherapy: Theory, Research & Practice, 15*(4), 314–317. 10.1037/h0086020

Chapter 8

The emotional performance

In addition to the therapist's practical expertise, we must take into account the therapist's vivid emotional life, as it inevitably plays into their performance in the room. This emotionality can be unveiled anywhere from moments of countertransference, unintentional self-disclosures, understated facial expressions or pointed active listening, and it exists in every session with every patient. As Ralph Greenson says, the therapist's ability to tolerate both love and hate of the patient is a secret, painful burden they can never truly communicate (Aaron, 1974). A perpetual unconscious, id-driven telenovela of dramatic, outlandish proportions. That dynamic emotional world – the personality of passion – may sometimes duel with the therapist's other features. Or they may coalesce. Who's to say.

Emotions constantly exist alongside the therapist's ever-shifting, ever-evolving intrapsychic life, and they fold into the ways that they will react to and receive the content of the patient. The analytic tool used by therapists to practice is always influenced by, as Abend calls it, their "so-called normal personalities," including their so-called normal internal conflicts, histories, and acquaintance with strong feelings (1989). It's undeniable that therapists are drawn to the work because of familiar sentiments in their inner lives. "Those who have no choice but to be filled with emotion," Nancy McWilliams says, "may be attracted to psychoanalytic ideas because they give voice to our affectively suffused experience and help us to make sense of our intense, insistent inner lives" (2004). And becoming deeply entrenched in their work can become one of the most glamorous parts of doing therapy; one of McWilliams's students went so far as to say that she was a self-ascribed "affect junky," someone who thrives on the intense emotional experiences in the session (2004). And these moments, "both conscious and unconscious, intended and unintended, transference-based and real," all inform a therapist's identity (Levine, 2007).

To indulge in a moment of *déjà vu*, let's not forget our thesis statement. How a therapist's emotional performance relates to performance art is simple: the therapist ingests the carrots of emotion-laden experiences, digests them, and displays them in a way all their own. To see how this occurs, we continue

DOI: 10.4324/9781003412694-12

to languish over our long dinner, faced with a dish we eat often; emotion, something we all know very well. But now, we will have it in a deconstructed form. Now, we attempt to describe the emotional performance.

What is the emotional performance?

If the structural performance is the nuts and bolts of your practice, the recipe from which you build your favorite dish, the emotional performance are the ingredients you use. It is the fundamental pieces from which your practice's structure can be internalized or neglected, embraced or rejected, learned or ignored. Your past, your present, your weaknesses and strengths, empathy and disgust, insecurities and conflicts – these are all what your emotional performance is made of. It is the sum of what you feel, why you feel that way, and how that gets expressed in the session. And as these feelings are intrapsychic in nature, the defenses that cover them may facilitate or detract from your ability to form and maintain a structural performance; when they're buried and remain unspoken, they can cause substantial rifts in the therapeutic alliance and sometimes even drive patients away (Curran et al., 2019).

Beyond simply serving as a connecting factor, one that can bind a patient and therapist together in a cinematic moment of excitement, an emotional performance serves many purposes. Uncontrollable moments of instability, when addressed with mindfulness, are eventually channeled into helpful tools through a therapist's ever-evolving emotional intellect. By facing emotions rather than running from them, one can eventually leverage their own psyches without becoming hateful, hurtful, sadistic, or redirecting the session to focus on themselves. This utilization of the emotional performance binds therapists beyond their structural modalities; "experienced therapists of different persuasions are more similar to each other than are novices across different schools of thought" due to their abilities to modulating emotions and express them tactfully (Lazarus, 1978). Over time, the peaks and valleys of emotion that the therapist experiences throughout their work bind them to the zeitgeist of therapy to create a calm, cool, and collected clinician with confidence and clarity in the room.

Just as Marinetti declaimed as a way to provide "liberation" from an antiquated state of pacifism, the therapist too declaims with emotion when they see something of the norm within the patient that brings about a powerful urge to change the status quo. Declaiming; to speak "bombastically," "to recite something as an exercise in elocution" (Merriam-Webster, n.d.). Declaiming includes the eventual attempt to persuade or empower, to stand on your soapbox and be heard for even a moment. Sometimes, the therapist encounters some stimuli that enlivens them, and they feel (consciously or unconsciously) that they must stand on their soapbox and be heard. This is the emotional performance of the therapist – the human element – the cry of personhood.

How does the emotional performance look?

How emotional performance articulates itself and takes root varies for every therapist with every patient each and every day. Like one's adherence to a particular theoretical model, it ebbs and flows, and the moment dictates the appropriate reaction. But unlike the structural performance, the "mistakes" in execution aren't so cut and dry. The therapist simply cannot avoid being a participant in the therapy, as they are the ones asking questions that stir up fantasies and reactions in all parties (Blatt & Behrends, 1987). Some may even go so far as to say that true neutrality (or rather, subjectivity) is unachievable due to the intensity of these emotions – ones that swirl around the therapist's internal world and the patient's (Renick, 1993). The way the therapist feels and the way they act can sometimes be at odds. But as long as a patient isn't being hurt or damaged, the internal experience of emotion can be an incredibly powerful tool. In fact, the stronger the countertransference reaction, the more important the topic is to work through healthily (Maroda, 1991).

To a psychoanalytic ear, this all sounds like countertransference. But in the emotional performance, countertransference is only one piece of the puzzle. The four main features of the emotional performance that we'll outline here are *personal ethics, countertransference, empathy,* and *impulsivity.* In the same way that we used Freudian techniques to explore potential structural performances, we'll do the same with these qualities. However, this is by no means an exhaustive list, and the thoughtful diner that you are, I'm sure you'll think of more on your own.

One's *personal ethics* are a system of beliefs one holds outside the therapy room which sometimes elicits strong emotional reactions. These beliefs could be moral, ethical, or concerning the fundamental ways humans treat one another. Examples would be a therapist who feels outrage hearing of a gay patient's homophobic parent, sadness hearing of a patient who experienced abuse from a partner, or disgust at a patient who previously embezzled from their place of work – a case of who's "good" and "bad." These cases chip away at a therapist's inner sense of morality like tapping at the hard shell of a crème brûlée – eventually, the gooey, emotional reactions beneath will ooze to the surface, and you cannot control from which cracks they emerge or to where they might ooze. The content or outcome of the situation itself is even sometimes a red herring, as "even ordinary normal morality has a harshly restraining, cruelly prohibiting quality" due to the unconscious conflicts that surround it (Freud, 1923). One's personal ethics coming into the room can look like unconsciously influencing a patient to make certain decisions (Hoffer, 1994) or lending positive regard to a patient that scratches a particular moral itch for the therapist.

The emotional component of various ethical situations, such as abuse or neglect, is not to be confused with the actual obligations of the therapist.

As a mandated reporter in serious cases of potential or ongoing violence, the ethics of the job become less like moral logic problems and more like situations that pride survival over all else. This is how having personal ethics can aid a clinician's treatment. They also enforce proper boundaries by working as an internal barometer of appropriate behavior, serving as a superego to your very practice at large. But beneath the more useful aspects of one's personal ethics lies the therapist's inner life, which emerges with the right pretense and opens feelings in the therapist about topics that they perhaps have not worked out on their own. For instance, "this patient's outrage about being caught for something unethical feels *wrong* to me" or "the world has socialized this patient's demographic *badly*." Personal moral and ethical imperatives are complicated, dependent on one's culture, one's upbringing, their experiences, and their relationships. Trust and rapport are established when a therapist views the patient as "a moral agent" on their own, utilizing their own moral agency to "inform [their] own behavior" rather than being "reduced to subjective opinion or attitude" (Gibson, 2005).

Next, there's *countertransference*, a well-tread topic in therapeutic literature. If a therapist has a certain association to a patient (for instance, if the patient reminds them of a parent, partner, friend, or past associate) there can be a litany of unconscious reactions that slip out at any given moment. Even the seemingly cold and unfeeling therapist of yore experienced countertransference reactions, as it's built into the process of therapy (Heimann, 1950). The fundamental difference between countertransference and personal ethics is that countertransferences are about *people* and personal ethics are about *concepts*. Sometimes they overlap, as is expected in deeply complex relationships. And as all therapists know, while rogue countertransference can cause problems, well-utilized countertransference is like a good roux for a mac'n'cheese; adding body and dimension to the treatment.

Abend (1989) reminds us that Freud identified transference in the patient in two categories – neurotic transferences and "benign, useful" transferences – and that the therapist's countertransference can be conceptualized in the same way. He continues that a therapist might gratify wishes that the patient is unconsciously seeking or the therapist might be reacting to the patient's similarity to a key figure in their lives. The therapist's countertransference, Abend continues, is a necessary part of the treatment, as it can reflect notions that the patient may be concealing (1989). Using it to a therapist's advantage, almost strategically and insightfully, can aid the treatment immensely.

Empathy is the next feature of the emotional performance, and boy, is it a great one. The act of empathy involves relating to, identifying with, and feeling for a patient, all while expressing it in adherence with your theoretical modality. Wild and scandalous for the time, Heinz Kohut was a paragon of integrating it into psychoanalytic technique. Empathy is key for the Kohutian therapist, as it "allows first for a therapeutic alliance to form ...

as therapy progresses, empathy allows the patient to look beyond what the therapist can offer" (McLean, 2007). Empathy isn't about being liked, admired, or appreciated by the patient; they simply seek to relate, and allow for their empathetic immersion, which is inevitably a long-term process, to inform the treatment.

In Kohut's groundbreaking lecture, "On empathy," he mentions a session in which he is seeing a woman on the brink of suicide. He says to her, "How would you feel if I let you hold my fingers, for a little while now while you are talking" – "I am not recommending it," he tells the audience, "But I was desperate. I was deeply worried" (1981). Some say that the duel-edged sword of empathy can be seen here; rather than enabling the patient's discomfort, his comments or actions served as an attempt to contain her unruly, terrifying, and destructive feelings. Holding a hand could be comparable to throwing a wet towel over a campfire instead of than allowing it to burn out on its own, dissolving the logs of conflict beneath it – something his structurally psychoanalytic training would have taught him. But the emotional performance overtook Kohut's structural performance in that moment, and everything turned out alright; a triumph for empathy!

And finally, a therapist's *impulsivity* should speak for itself, as an emotional performance can be influenced by how viscerally one reacts to stimuli. The impulsive reply in question could be anger – a therapist who gets angry and puts that anger on display – but it isn't limited to angry outbursts. We could also see sadness, entertainment, disbelief, or any other emotion. Studies show that therapy can be harmful for clients who experience therapists to be emotionally reactive, triggering intense feelings in both parties without meaningful resolutions (Curran et al., 2019, Lilienfeld, 2007). Additionally, emotional reactivity reframes the session around the therapist's feelings, and the patient begins to feel responsible for moderating or withholding potentially pertinent information about their lives for the sake of avoiding the therapist's perceived wrath. And though it might seem outlandish, there are benefits to the occasional dalliance with impulsivity – benefits we'll see in how technique becomes performance. In fact, it can be something of a necessity for certain kinds of emotional performance.

How emotion becomes skill: From performance into technique

Turning a structural performance into a structural technique involves integrating knowledge into an individualized modus operandi – following the recipe and baking your own cake. However, turning emotional performance into emotional technique can, in some ways, be a different animal. While both take time, energy, a degree of humility, and a lot of mindfulness, utilizing emotions in the service of someone else takes a certain kind of insight into oneself to know *when* emotions are being had, *what* those emotions might be, and *why* they might be popping up. Additionally, emotional performances can be used in conjunction with structural performances or in direct opposition to them. If one has been taught throughout their schooling to remain as neutral as possible, and yet they find themselves rolling their eyes, sighing exasperatedly, or clearing their throat in indignation, they might not be adhering to their neutral stance so well.

Emotional performances that work in tandem with structural performances are what one would consider a certain kind of "technique," as even one's feelings (however sudden and powerful they might be) can be leveraged into the treatment thoughtfully with an amount of insight. Think of Kohut's hand-holding – he outrightly says that he wouldn't recommend it to anyone, but it fits within the structure of his practice (in which the building blocks are empathy, positive regard, and togetherness). The main difference between an emotional performance and an outburst isn't always the moment of emotion itself. While not all emotional performances need to be clearly delineated from structural ones, for the purposes of illuminating how it looks in its purest form, we'll be talking about a certain kind of emotional performance that's reflective of the sometimes off-the-cuff nature of therapy. This, a pure emotional performance, is a mix of *the incident of emotion* and how that emotion is picked apart *after the incident*.

First, we'll talk about how the moment of emotion: *the incident of emotion*. A horrifying thought! While it might make a traditional analyst cringe, there are times that a therapist may become swept up in emotion towards a patient, which results in reactivity – or, the puzzle piece we spoke of before, *impulsivity*. This is where impulsivity has merit; many times, it is the way an emotional performance emerges, as it is a natural eschewing of structural technique. A supervisor[1] was once hosting a group supervision where a budding Masters of Social Work (MSW) informed her peers that she frequently responds to a patient's query of "how are you?" with "I'm absolutely exhausted." The supervisor responded that whether the therapist knows it or not, this is an emotional reply – which could be perhaps even considered a narcissistic or a sadistic acting out – that unconsciously relays to the patient that they're a burden on the therapist's packed schedule. Even if the emotions are authentic to the therapist, they're still being displayed in the session in a particular tenor and register, dripping with latent content. Here, saying "I'm absolutely exhausted" is the emotional incident.

Emotional incidents in the session can also manifest more explosively, such as Mitchell's idea of a "therapeutic outburst" (Mitchell, 1997). In this situation, a therapist lays it all on the table in terms of affect, expressing deep thoughts or feelings to a patient – an Oscar-winning performance, for sure. Despite potential discomfort at the initial onset of the denouement, a therapeutic outburst ideally ends in a cinematic moment of renewal and growth between the two; "the therapist fears having made things worse, only to discover that it actually made things better, even if it scared the patient a little"

(Maroda, 1995). While sometimes these moments can be messier or more painful than a good episode of "*In Treatment*" or "*Couples Therapy,*" the end result is something cathartic and beautiful. Like Carl Rogers sucking on a cigarette after the Gloria session, your sleeves rolled up and your tie loose, you bask in the feeling of a risk paid off.

Then, of course, comes the complicated matter of *processing these incidences.* This follow-up is what turns an organic moment of fervency into something that's valuable for helping the patient. Bringing these moments to light can be difficult, especially when coping with a therapist's statements which could have impacted the therapeutic alliance. Tolpin (Aaron, 1974) argued that these little waves of emotion are a route to explore new ideas in the treatment, as they fuel self-observation. Much like one would be inquisitive about a patient's visceral reaction to a topic, one must be inquisitive about their own, as it illuminates certain emotional riddles yet unsolved about the case and oneself. Van Leewen (Aaron, 1974) argues that countertransference is an excellent barometer to nuclear conflicts in both parties (or in the alliance itself). So while they're difficult, and sometimes excruciating to process, they can ultimately benefit everyone involved as long as the follow-up is handled with care, dignity, communication, and compassion. The one thing that these emotional performances never lack is meaning, as there's no such thing as a "reasonable response" to a patient's material that doesn't require further introspection (Abend, 2018). Evaluating these reactions is absolutely critical to the work.

A lovely and succulent course – and now, we're all done. We've got a rough idea of how an emotional performance works in a vacuum. And we've got a rough idea of how a structural performance works in a vacuum as well. But what do these two performances look like together – and how do they create the identity of the *performance therapist?* I hope you're still hungry, as we've got lots more to do.

Note

1   Who wishes to remain anonymous, lest he become a former supervisor.

References

Aaron, R. (1974). The analyst's emotional life during work. *Journal of the American Psychoanalytic Association, 22,* 160–169.

McWilliams, N. (2004). *Psychoanalytic psychotherapy: A practitioner's guide.* New York: The Guilford Press.

Levine, S.S. (2007). Nothing but the truth: Self-disclosure, self-revelation, and the persona of the analyst. *Journal of the American Psychoanalytic Association, 55,* 81–104.

Curran, J., Parry, G.D., Hardy, G.E., Darling, J., Mason, A.M., & Chambers, E. (2019). How does therapy harm? A model of adverse process using task analysis in the meta-synthesis of service users' experience. *Frontiers in psychology, 10,* 347. 10.3389/fpsyg.2019.00347

Lazarus, A. (1978). Style not systems. *Psychotherapy: Theory, Research and Practice, 15,* 359–361.

Merriam-Webster. (n.d.). Declaim. In Merriam-Webster.com dictionary. Retrieved November 11, 2022, from https://www.merriam-webster.com/dictionary/declaim

Blatt, S.J., & Behrends, R.S. (1987). Internalization, separation-individuation, and the nature of therapeutic action. *International Journal of Psychoanalysis, 68,* 279–297.

Renik, O. (1993). Analytic interaction: Conceptualizing technique in light of the analyst's irreducible subjectivity. *Psychoanalytic Quarterly, 62,* 553–571.

Freud, S. (1923). The ego and the id. In J. Strachey et al. (Trans.), *The standard edition of the complete psychological works of Sigmund Freud,* Volume XIX (pp. 1–66). London: Hogarth Press.

Hoffer, A. (1994). The development of psychoanalysis by Sándor Ferenczi and Otto Rank (1924). *Journal of the American Psychoanalytic Association, 42*(3), 851–862. 10.1177/000306519404200309

Gibson S. (2005). On judgment and judgmentalism: How counselling can make people better. *Journal of Medical Ethics, 31,* 575–577.

Heimann, P. (1950). On counter-transference. *International Journal of Psychoanalysis, 31,* 81–84.

Abend, S.M. (1989). Countertransference, empathy, and the analytic ideal: The impact of life stresses on analytic capability. *Psychoanalytic Quarterly, 55*(4), 563–575.

McLean, J. (2007). Psychotherapy with a narcissistic patient using kohut's self psychology model. *Psychiatry (Edgmont (Pa.: Township), 4*(10), 40–47. Retrieved from https://www.ncbi.nlm.nih.gov/pmc/articles/PMC2860525/

Kohut. (1981). In Ornstein P. (Ed.), The search for the self: Selected writings of Heinz Kohut. London: Karnac Books. Republished in 2011.

Lilienfeld, S.O. (2007). Psychological treatments that cause harm. *Perspectives on Psychological Science, 2*(1), 53–70. 10.1111/j.1745-6916.2007.00029.x

Abend, S.M. (1989). Countertransference and psychoanalytic technique. *Psychoanalytic Quarterly, 58*(3), 374–395.

Mitchell, S.A. (1997). *Influence and autonomy in psychoanalysis* (1st ed.). Routledge. 10.4324/9781315803326

Maroda, K. (1995). Projective identification and countertransference interventions: Since feeling is first. *Psychoanalytic Review, 82,* 229–247.

Maroda, K. (1991). *The power of the countertransference: Innovations in analytic technique.* London, England: John Wiley and Sons.

Chapter 9

The intersection of structure and emotion

How a therapeutic performance looks

All these ideas about theory and emotion in a therapist's performance can certainly make for a thought-provoking menu. But what of eating? There exists a realm between stoic intellectualism and outbursts of reactivity that adds some complicated, complex flavors into the therapeutic stew, flavors you can't quite taste just by looking at a description of the dish. It's not as simple as combining "learned practical" knowledge with "implicit emotional" knowledge; the ingredients are organic, artisan, bespoke – you've met the goats that made the cheese, you've grown the carrots in your own backyard garden – and there are strong influences of your personal past and present in every drop. When the elements of structural performance and emotional performance come together, we create something called the *therapeutic performance* – a way that the performance therapist is or isn't in session.

As the two forces of emotional performance and theoretical performance are both incessantly in play for the therapist, there must be a way for them to coexist. A therapist recognizing the role of their own ego strengths and weaknesses might sound familiar to the relational therapist. However, just to nip this academic note in the bud before we go any further, I'll address what more theory-versed readers have probably been wondering for some time; the performance therapist (and the therapeutic performance) is not a relational argument. While relationalists might think of the model of the performance therapist as a synonym for countertransference – the reactions, the thoughts, the theoretical knowledge, and integration – it's simply their theoretical frame that provides a preexisting catch-all for terms also used here. The claim of the performance therapist is that this genuine relationship does not come from the theoretical standpoint, or even the personal authenticity of the therapist, but the delicate combination of the two. From a relational perspective, the therapist's relationship directly with the patient is usually the key that unearths drives and motives, which isn't at all what the above is suggesting. Instead, in a broader sense, this idea of the therapist is more about how natural humanity can be leveraged in cultivating a therapeutic identity.

DOI: 10.4324/9781003412694-13

As we attempt to understand how a therapeutic performance looks with all its working parts, we run into a bit of a problem: our guest of honor. Let us revisit the idea of the Jungian persona; the imago of an ideal therapist that many practitioners seek to emulate (or repudiate). The Jungian persona is a thing that chooses "various roles, integrating them more or less into the dominant ego-identity" as we attempt to nurture our "developing egos" (Hall, 1983). And this ideal delivers a "vital sector of the personality which provides the individual with a container, a protective covering for his or her inner self" (Hopcke, 1989). The persona is thought of as something outside of oneself – a part of something more profound, more historic, more ancestral, less internal. Often, performance artists execute their pieces believing that they're communicating a message that's bigger than just themselves. The persona is the mask they don, ornamented with culture, politics, antiquity, or whatever else they are attempting to communicate. And a therapist looking to ease the pain of the patient, the person they have made a vow to help, feels they must don the same kind of mask–that of the Ideal Therapist–to get the job done.

The attempt at recognizing, addressing, and integrating the persona of the Ideal Therapist can quickly go awry. An accurate assessment of this nebulous, forceful persona is that it's just an idyllic fantasy. This brilliant character, the humble expert, is read about in books (Yalom, 1989), seen them on tape (Shostrom, 1965), or heard them speak in interviews (Puder, 2023). A supervisor, a professor, a friend, someone you follow on Twitter, your own therapist; whoever you may admire and praise, that is the image that haunts your mind, the unreachable aspiration of a perfect clinician. A silent, watchful parent. A nurturing yet strict, compassionate, empathetic yet grounding observer. One whose structure is solid and whose emotions are well-communicated. A countertransference-free being of pure curiosity. You hate them, you love them, you wish you were them. You never will be.

The Ideal Therapist has certainly shifted over the years, and there is no longer one tweed-suited, bespectacled, bearded septuagenarian that's universally accepted as the blueprint. In modernity, the Ideal Therapist looks different in the many circles of therapy that exist now. The Ideal EMDR Practitioner is quite unalike from the Ideal Analyst, and the Ideal TikTok Mental Health Counselor is an entirely different cuisine than the Ideal Private Practitioner Who Does Not Take Insurance. One could say that the vision of the perfect therapist, one who everyone attempts to live up to, is different depending on who you're asking. But there are certain archetypes influenced by culture that weasel their way into the general consciousness of helpless therapists who get a great deal of exposure to these characters. The more analytic trainings one attends, the more they'll imagine that being the Ideal Therapist means letting the patient guide the treatment. And the more compassion-focused therapy (CFT) groups one visits, the more they'll imagine that the Ideal Therapist activates the patient's parasympathetic nervous system with ease.[1]

Largely, the prevalent version of the Ideal Therapist is immensely over-whelming to live up to. Whereas Ideal [Successful] Therapists of yesteryear were also academics, scholars, and writers, therapists in the present day have to be the best at marketing, public relations, social media content creation, billing, business-owning, navigating technology, and on top of everything, networking with others who also wish to be the Ideal Therapist (how gru-eling!). They must be someone who propagates and lives by a message of social justice both in and out of the session, and prides themselves on being non-judgmental, inclusive, and open-minded (NASW, 2021). The more certificates, the better the Ideal Therapist is at therapy – weekend seminars and the latest acronyms are his bread and butter to "increase [his] marketability" (Clay, 2010). Social media is a buzz with one therapist's tips to another, with quotes from writers and speakers, with clinicians offering mental health advice to both patients and non-patients *en masse* (Kolmes, 2012). The modern therapist, the Ideal Therapist, has more pots on the stove than any other therapist before him – and he's expected to handle them with ease.

To assume a deeply impersonal and unreasonable expectation, comparing oneself to this pure, unsoiled, supreme figure, is incredibly unrealistic for the burgeoning therapist. It almost removes responsibility one has to work to-wards cultivating their own identities, and instead, twists their conceptions of a good therapist into a persona rife with conflict. In the attempt to remember all the moving parts of their performance – so many structures, so many emotions – their therapeutic performance morphs into a litany of dis-placements and projections. It becomes a way to imagine one is working towards self-actualization by maintaining the illusion that they're building towards a therapeutic ideal. Perhaps, in a way, the attempt to live as a persona eventually becomes synthesized into one's work ego, thereby transforming it into an idealized image. But in reality, this therapist is *acting* as a surgeon without *being* a surgeon to defend against feelings of inadequacy. As for why one might fall into this cycle, it's inadvisable to generalize. But if we look back at Horney, we can take a guess: holding oneself up to an unattainable standard allows someone to reject themselves rather than experiencing the painful, uncertain surprise of being rejected by others.

And there we have the therapeutic performance. A wickedly difficult act complicated by contemporariness and muddled by insecurity. The perform-ance therapist exists to reflect the world around him, just as the performance artist does. And sadly, it's a convoluted world. However, a glimmer of hope lies in the shining eyes of our guest of honor – for every persona, individuation is possible. While the primary phase in the metamorphosis of the performance therapist is to see the Ideal Therapist and begin to emulate him, there is still a long journey ahead. In a teenage rebellion, the secondary phase is where the therapist begins to become. Their performance slips out in bits and pieces, showing signs of integration and flashes of relaxation. In an unconscious attempt to assert individuality against a persona that feels oppressive, the undoing begins as conscious and unconscious emotional performances occur. As is the eternal balance of the psyche, one is always fighting with and against oneself – to be or not to be the Ideal Therapist. And finally, moments of individuation occur in the final stage as the performance therapist is comfortable enough to learn, feel, take in, and express. And though individuation is never static, and performances change throughout life due to one's emotional and intellectual evolution, therapy begins to feel less like a family business one inherited from an expectant parent and more like a restaurant one built themselves.

Another place setting is in order

Now that we have a good sense of how one eats carrots, the various types, the techniques of mastication and numerous flavor profiles, now we can really take a bite, and see how each of these facets looks on the therapeutic stage. Performing in the therapeutic frame isn't necessarily a theatrical feat, and sometimes, it can be quite mundane. Not every performance is one that presents as falsely dramatic or excessively expressive – not every False Self has a feather boa. But regardless of how your defenses present, there are ways that a therapist enters into a performance of sorts; the spirit of the act takes over, just as it does with the patient – and both enter into a scene without narrative, a dialogue without a script. You're attempting to balance whichever persona, self-state, work ego, or idealized image you put on that morning with whatever feelings are underneath. And the thing that threatens to crack your facade isn't yourself. It's the other person sitting in the room with you.

If it isn't enough for the therapist to have their own structural performance, emotional performance, and identity (as we spoke of in Part II) – this table is reserved for a party of two, not one. The therapeutic performance isn't just in a therapists' ability to "act like" a therapist or integrate their act into their personhood, as the therapy room is not a vacuum. Instead of the therapist taking a pair of scissors and snipping a piece of their own hair off, the patient has the scissors, snipping and slicing and stabbing as they will as the therapist attempts to receive the onslaught with the silent acknowledgment that it is their duty to do so (Abramović, 1974). Both find themselves in enactments and repetitions, posturing and regressing, reflecting, and pontificating – a *performance á deux*. Essentially, therapy is an "interaction between two personalities ... each personality has its internal and external dependencies, anxieties, and pathological defenses", and though the therapist presents in technique and form as a less impulsively responsive force, "each of these whole personalities ... responds to every event of the analytic situation" (Racker, 1988).

Whether intentional or unintentional, performative, reactive, or both, the way that the performance looks in session constantly serves as a way of transmuting, defending against, and voicing unconscious fantasies. To Aron and Atlas, these "dramatic dialogues" were ways that the therapeutic dyad articulates and engages with both parties' numerous self-states in psychic realms of dreaming, playing, repeating, and reacting (2017). To many others, this is the natural, inexplicable evolution of a therapy. And just as a small aside; as we talk about the patient and the therapist, it should be known that these two perspectives are *one in the same* – simply two sides to the same flapjack. A therapist can see a patient in themselves, and if a patient is also a therapist, it works the same way. There's no way to know if every therapist reading this work is in therapy themselves, but in a way, it's sort of presupposed. After all, therapy is the most effective way to learn about oneself. We would know, wouldn't we.

Though only the patient has the scissors in their hand, the therapist's flinching, sighing, or screaming (as they are wont to do) are all based on the pretext of the therapeutic situation. These micro-performances (reactions, exclamations, or withdrawals) are stirred on by the patient's prodding and are quite situational in nature. Perhaps they serve to protect or defend portions of the therapist's identity that they'd rather not expose, or perhaps they are ways of reacting with anger, ragefully fighting back against the beating they're being given. They remain a part of the performer's identity whether the performer wants them to be seen or not – so let's explore them next.

Note

1   This is very lightly paraphrased from interviews and only confirmed with a quick Google search, so I acknowledge it may be off base; my hours of research were spent on other topics.

References

Hall. (1983). *Jungian dream interpretation: A handbook of theory and practice.* Toronto, Ontario: Inner City Books.

Hopcke. (1989). *A guided tour of the collected works of C. G. Jung.* Boulder, Colorado: Shambhala. Republished in 2013.

National Association of Social Workers (NASW). (2021). *Code of ethics.* Washington, DC. Web. https://www.socialworkers.org/About/Ethics/Code-of-Ethics/Code-of-Ethics-English

Clay, R. (2010). Gaining specialty certification. *American Psychological Association.* American Psychological Association, https://www.apa.org/gradpsych/2010/03/specialty-certification.

Kolmes, K. (2012). Social media in the future of professional psychology. *Professional Psychology: Research and Practice, 43*(6), 606–612. 10.1037/a0028678

Abramović. (1974). *Rhythm 0 [performance].* Naples, Italy: Studio Morra.

Racker, H. (1988). Transference and countertransference. *The international psycho-analytical library* (pp. 1–196). London, UK: The Hogarth Press. Web.

Aron, L., & Atlas, G. (2017). Dramatic dialogue: Dreaming & drama in contemporary clinical practice. *Psychoanalytic Perspectives, 16.* Web.

Puder, M. (Host). (2023, March 3). Nancy McWilliams on Mental Health, Transference and Dissociation (Ep. 171) [Audio podcast episode]. In *Psychiatry & Psychotherapy Podcast.* https://www.psychiatrypodcast.com/psychiatry-psychotherapy-podcast/episode-171-nancy-mcwilliams-on-mental-health-transference-and-dissociation

Shostrom, E. (Director). (1965). *Three approaches to psychotherapy* [Film]. Psychological Films Inc.

Yalom, I. (1989). Love's Executioner. Basic Books.New York City: NY.

Chapter 10

The therapeutic table set for two

Built into the invariable structures of two humans interacting with one another in this specific set of circumstances comes an expressive connection that exists in layers and nuance (whether openly discussed in a palpable way or symbolically in a philosophical one). This connection is called the *transference space*, where a patient treats the therapist like their parents, their lovers, their siblings, friends, mentors, adversaries, and everything in between. It is a place where forbidden emotions can be expressed, where fantasies of relationships play out, where the patient is able to transform the therapist into whoever they may consciously or unconsciously choose. A therapist's reactions to a patient's transference, whether they're forthright or subtle, are some of the most powerful tools available in the therapy. They tangle in this interplay – the patient has some sort of transference reaction, the therapist responds in a certain way (perhaps a countertransference reaction!), and the two turn this complicated back-and-forth into something that aids in reducing symptoms, enhancing relationships, and embracing self-realization. Seems easy enough, no?

If the therapist is the performance artist in this scenario, the patient is everything else: their counterpart, their biggest critic, their most ardent supporter, their sponsor, their fascination, their repulsion, their partner, and enemy. Into the transference space, the patient brings their carrots – but they have trouble making sense of the things. And so, they give them to the therapist, the one who will take them in and give them back in a new form. In their execution of the carrot-eating (the very performance of therapy itself!), the therapist might have an idea of what they're trying to communicate, but that's not always the case. Sometimes, the communication is dominated by structure; a polite meal with copious amounts of intellectual insight and no elbows on the table. Sometimes, emotion is at the forefront, and the performance is bizarre, animalistic, so very human. Carrots are flying, saliva is everywhere, everyone is feeling sick, dirty, and they can't look away. And once the therapist begins to develop their orange glow, the interpretation of this performance is done with curiosity (ideally, anyway, lest their own defenses deny them the opportunity for growth). But let's break it down even further.

DOI: 10.4324/9781003412694-14

How the structural performance looks in the transference space is quite different depending on how the therapist has been trained to view transference. Some schools of thought say that positive transference should be thought of as a direct route to healing (Welling, 2018) while other modalities believe that unanalyzed negative transference can result in an odd form of dependency on the therapist (Greenacre, 1954). Either way, everyone's unique training makes for a state fair with a table full of distinct cherry pies. That being said, a similarity that all therapists have despite their varied training (or perhaps because of it) is in the creation of a genuine relationship with the patient using whatever techniques might be at their disposal. And every genuine relationship, even those outside the frame, have glimmers of transference be they positive or negative – transference that needs to be addressed with skill, lest the therapist gets sucked into the patient's vortex unknowingly (Andersen & Przybylinski, 2012).

Now, is a relationship in the transference space "genuine" in the sense that both parties are wholly invested in the same way? Old school therapists would say not, and they have a point. Rather than seeing the therapist as a whole object, when the transference is thick and dense and permeates the entire session, the patient has trouble seeing them as anything other than the parts they can make out through the haze (Hayman, 1990). These parts resemble transference objects of their youth (primary caregivers in particular), and it takes a while for the patient to see through this mirage and connect with the therapist for who they really are rather than what they represent (Money-Kyrle, 1978; Ingram, 1993). The therapist, on the other hand, views it all – including whichever transference figure the patient may be confusing them for. And therein lies the structural performance in the transference; to use the genuine relationship they're forming with the patient to help them see as well.

The emotional performance in the transference space is also highly individualized, but more so about the therapist's nature (though their training does play a part in molding that nature). The therapist is invited to the patient's dinner party, but when they arrive, the house is dark, and the patrons are groping around, looking for light. Much like the Charcot's hysteric patients fumbled about in a hazy pantomime, their graphic theatrics conveying feelings beyond words, so too does the therapist wander in the transference space, their emotional performance one of uncertainty and fervor. Fumbling in the dark, they find themselves rooms with names like "role responsiveness," "defenses," "repetitions," "displacements" – and with no light, they cannot see what they've gotten themselves into. All the while, the patient frequently confuses them for their primary caregivers, their relationship partners, or their other close contacts. It is thrilling, scary, irritating, rigorous, sometimes insipid, eventful and uneventful. All these dinner parties in the dark, the therapist says, and so much time looking for light switches! Will we ever eat?

These many aspects of transference, these "rooms," all have shades of performance, as they're loaded with emotion that the therapist must modulate and express in ways commensurate with their training. But of transference's many gradations, there are two that fit well into the model of the performance therapist, as they very plainly walk identity's thin tightrope of performance and the self that lies beneath it. They are *acting out* and *enactments*. While these two concepts share certain characteristics, there is one main difference: acting out is perpetrated from one party to the other party while an enactment is a scene in which two people get caught up in specific roles that one may unconsciously be pulling from the other. More simply put: enactments are a lunch date for two – reservations made in advance – and acting out is one person giving another a pie in the face.

The act of "acting out"

One of the most relevant pieces of transference within the conversation on performance is acting out – a literal "acting" of the id. Despite years of debate and development from Anna Freud to Phyllis Greenacre, the psychoanalytic community is coming close to a mutually agreeable definition of acting out (though don't count your chickens). Acting out, in somewhat rudimentary terms, is about how internal conflicts, fantasies, defenses, and general machinations are externalized in the session. Like the transference, acting out is a kind of "dramatized" resistance (Auchincloss, 2012). In acting out, the patient fears that the therapist sees them as a chef sees a deliciously large lobster; ready to boil alive and pick apart. The patient panics and snaps at the person they believe wants to do them harm. But unlike the lobster, the patient is at no risk of being eaten – even so, the fear is real, and they feel like they must fight for their lives. This can cause acting out to sometimes seem vicious and malicious. And even if tensions don't rise to that dramatic of a denouement, acting out serves to manage all kinds of anxiety, cull split-off parts of one's personality, and stave away potentially painful feelings.

In many ways, acting out allows one to perform fantasies, wishes, and fears – all a part of the id, which emerges with a kick like a bit too much cayenne in your bell pepper soup. For the most part, a patient doesn't deliberately intend to act out [though as with everything, there are always exceptions, as even hysterics of yore reportedly acted out symptoms for secondary gains (Lothane, 1995)]. They provoke and prod, pick up the scissors and snip away at the therapists' clothes, all sorts of inflammatory or outlandish embodiments of emotion to elicit some sort of reaction. Whether these drives are integrated into your identity or not, the act of acting out taps into the pleasure of wish fulfillment felt by the id. Interestingly, Lothane (2009, 2011) points out that Breuer and Freud used a German term for "acting out" that one would also use when describing the acting in a stage play. One could assume that this reflects the kind of performative nature of an act-out – that consciously or unconsciously, it exists to convey a message loud and clear for the patient to hear – *get me away from the transference* (Freud, 1905)!

The lesser-known version of acting out is called acting-in. Rather than acting in opposition to the transference in an attempt to avoid it, someone acts *with* the transference in an attempt to quell tension within it. It works the same way as acting out to "expel psychic reality," as "the function of communication contained in action" is rendered "overshadowed by its expulsive aim" – if the therapist is busy paying attention to this, one's unconscious mind thinks, they'll completely forget about the uncomfortable topic we've been exploring recently (Green, 1975). For example, if the therapy is beginning to confront a patient's idealized image of themselves as a strong-willed person, they may feel unconsciously driven to start an arbitrary argument with the therapist just to feel like they're not getting soft.

Acting out is not reserved specifically for the patient, though it's slightly less explored from the perspective of the therapist. Auchincloss & Samberg add that the therapist's "unconscious expression of countertransference" leads to acting out just like an unconscious expression of transference would (2012). Just like the various ways the patient would act out, the therapist, afraid of being boiled, shelled, and dipped in garlic butter, could be unconsciously motivated to come late, attempt to change the relationship with the patient, or in the worst cases, try to drive the patient to termination. Annie Reich (1951) added to this idea by explaining that acting out is an outcropping of countertransference, and consequently, one does not exist without the other. She posits that when a therapist becomes so focused on a patient's content as a way to avoid looking inside themselves at their own potential discomfort, they might hyper-focus on issues less relevant to the patient and more relevant to the therapist. In emphasizing conflicts in a way that over-inflates their importance, to Reich, the therapist is acting out to avoid their own countertransference. In Freud's words, "the greater the resistance, the more extensively will acting out (repetition) replace remembering" (1914). And in the words of the classic meme, "*I pretend I do not see it*" (Reactions, 2019).

Like any instance of countertransference, acting out doesn't have to be an explosive incident, and sometimes, the tiniest occurrences the most consistently feel like torture by a thousand cuts. The emotional performance of an act-out (or act-in) is always in the service of upholding a defense. So, while the feelings one might experience as a result of their act-out might be intense and destabilizing, they're also a displacement, used as a delicious red herring that distracts you from the meat and potatoes of the real issue. The countertransference that's being avoided may even be a stronger feeling, a more complicated one, a more agonizing one; one that directly confronts the aforementioned self that lies beneath what one believes their therapeutic performance to be.

While acting out might seem like a primarily emotional process, the structural performance is still present in a few ways. When a patient is acting out, they engage in behavior that they may or may not be privy to, and sometimes, the reasoning behind this behavior comes weeks or months after the incident itself. But for the therapist, someone tasked to maintain the frame by way of their structural knowledge, tolerating acting out is part of the performance of being a therapist. "There is nothing more surprising both to the patient and to the analyst than the revelations that occur in these moments of acting out," say Abram & Hjulmand, but "there must always follow a putting into words of the new bit of understanding." (1996). A structurally adept therapist (or at least one with curiosity trained into them) will be able to observe acting out on their part and assess how it plays into dynamics that were already present in the dyad.

And there we have one type of transference that the performance therapist must handle in their own way – in their cycle of metaphysical digestion, assimilation, and reflection. Now, let's have another.

The acting of enactments

Enactments are also a good example of a sort of complicated performance, one that can be anything from an intentional act of malice to the unintentional engagement in a pattern. But we run into a similar problem as we did with acting out – figuring out what the thing is in the first place. The definition of an enactment is so complicated that Bohleber and Fonagy [et al.] attempted to create a novella-length comprehensive definition for the term for the IPA Project Committee on Conceptual Integration (2013). Auchincloss & Samberg's seminal psychoanalytic glossary defines enactments as the interplay between the patient and the therapist when the realm of fantasy is transmuted into the session (2012), but what that looks like can vary based upon who you're asking. In some of the most traditional literature, the enactments of the therapist are beyond interpretation (in the therapy room, of course – they're free to interpret them in their own personal therapy all they want). And for others, therapist enactment can be sublimated into role play that will ultimately aid the patient in understanding past scenarios (Pagano, 2012). We see why Bohleber and Fonagy had their hands full.

Enactments range from the obvious to the subtle, the wild to the mundane, the confusing to the candid. But the problem with such a broad range of definitions is that enactments become both everything and nothing. Even something like a therapeutic alliance can be twisted into the patient seeking warmth from the therapist and the therapist reciprocating – an enactment to the tee (Stern, 2016). While taking enactments this seriously might seem a bit hyperbolic, it is in fact quite the serious issue; the French call enactments a *mise en acte*, like a *mise en scéne*, as it penetrates the very essence of the session (Bohleber et al., 2013). Two performers here, the patient and the therapist, engage in a dialogue as they perform for a rapt, invisible crowd. What is an enactment if not a repetition and recitation of lines learned over the course of one's life? Maybe they're not said verbatim, but the phrases and sentiments ring true once the enactment is in full swing. And what happens if the cyclical loop feels inescapable?

Handling enactments is difficult, primarily because a therapist can only notice and consider their enactments after the fact – such is the nature of the beast, as being in an enactment means being too emotionally involved to see outside the dynamic. Some see enactments as something avoidable, and consequently, "bad" for the therapist and the treatment. As they're defined mostly by the therapist's experience and training, it seems that any sort of action that can be perceived as stepping out of the traditional analytic method can be termed as an enactment, something as simple as commenting on a patient's appearance to proclaiming your deep hatred of a patient to their face. Others believe that in psychoanalytic psychotherapy, the therapist *has* to get emotionally involved "in a manner that he had not intended" for the treatment to be successful (Boesky, 1990). Browning (2016) tells readers an anecdote about reassuring a patient that they were beautiful – an enactment, but a helpful one nonetheless, as it assisted the patient in resolving lingering feelings about her father's view of her beauty. And this is truly why enactments are so complicated; while they can be seen as failures of structural performances, they can be successful emotional ones.

Emotional performance in the space of enactments can be some of the most volatile or intense moments in the session. Sometimes, the patient's carrots can be a bitter pill, and though they eventually show up on the therapist's skin, they feel pointed and suffocating. The therapist can't help but cough, choke, reach for their water – any reaction, sometimes without thinking. Like a patient acts out to protect themselves from harm, the therapist gets enmeshed in a psychic dynamic to unconsciously feed some fear, wish, or both. How often therapists feel themselves get bored, exhausted, overwhelmed, confused, depressed, angered, or thrilled by a patient. As soon as those emotions become visible in the session, they begin to serve a purpose for both parties. But when they continue uninterrupted and unanalyzed, as it may render the treatment less useful for the patient. As "fantasy is more primary than reality" in the session (Winnicott, 1945), even the faintest whiff of an enactment must be approached with curiosity, lest the remembering, repeating, and working through begins to cease.

Structural performance in the enactment space is tricky – some say it doesn't exist at all. Bohleber [et al.] point out that an enactment "involves the occurrence of something unexpected and thus incompatible with the relevant rules of therapeutic technique," because the therapist's "own vulnerability and personality enter directly into the treatment" (2013). However, technique and emotion can hardly be separated in this way – as we've learned, the vulnerability or personality, which certainly sound like two key qualities of the emotional performance, are integral to the performance therapist's process as well. Additionally, enactments are seen as a sort of "mistake" to many. Bohleber [et al.] described how some theorists believe that enactments are breakdowns in the therapist's supposed "normal" functioning as a therapist, as they indicate a "collapse" of theory that is overcome by emotion (2013). In some ways, this is true from a very rigid standpoint, as impulsivity from the therapist's perspective is in many ways contraindicated to the psychoanalytic process. But this ignores something very important: enactments aren't just moments of therapeutic weakness. They can often be rich and loaded with patterns of behavior that are sometimes recognizable or predictable, comparable to some kind of unconscious role play informed by the patient's content. In some ways, the therapist is drawing on these elements of presence and engagement that Karbelnig (2018) describes as necessary characteristics for their performance. As we've said before, with any relationship comes transference. So it stands to reason that getting lost in the relationship in a way that eventually facilitates transference (no matter the form) can be seen as something neither bad nor good – it's just a sign that the process is going as expected.

Additionally, if one does subscribe to the notion that enactments are blunders, the structural performance is there to make meaning from what can feel like chaos. It is a soft focaccia that mops up the remaining hollandaise sauce of the emotional performance once you've picked up the eggs Benedict and thrown them against the wall. Once the therapist is able to use the technique they're been trained in to recognize how they fell into the enactment and why it happened, the relationship can progress. So, by utilizing skill that addresses, acknowledges, and appreciates some of the more difficult feelings in the moment of enacting, the therapist and patient can clean their plates and ready themselves for the next course – or rather, the next stage of their therapeutic alliance.

Someone call the waiter

Here we reach the end of our third course, and as we conclude, we see a sort of philosophical problem highlighted by the performance therapist's handling of the transference space. Handling either transference or countertransference, be it through enactments, acting out, or anything else, means simultaneously being aware of one's emotions and leveraging them in a way that ensures their usefulness. That being said, being open to this kind of insight and preparedness can sometimes be uncomfortable for many therapists, who might believe themselves to be manipulative (Boesky, 1990). One of the stated goals of the performance therapist (more of which we'll get into later)[1] is to utilize one's personhood to aid in the healing and development of their patients – this personhood being everything structural, such as training, experience, schooling, and the like, along with everything emotional, like one's history, personal emotional growth, and willingness to empathize or relate. Performance, performance, performance, we say – it seems to be all about the performance. But if we're in a continual conversation about the difference between one's external self and their internal selves, that brings to light the question: is the therapist rendered *inauthentic* if they employs their person-hood like a tool? When the inner self is externalized with intent, does it stop being genuine?

A controversial yet true statement is that, alas, the therapist themselves is but a person, and potentially even a patient themselves at one point; someone with conflicts and resolutions, trauma and triumph. Consequently, they too have within them this elusive concept called selfhood, which we went over pretty thoroughly in Part II. That selfhood was then worked out and extra-polated here into a therapeutic identity – a therapeutic performance. Then, we added the patient, which brings the identity of the performance therapist out of conjecture an into reality. But in some ways, it feels like we've made the pastry shell, but have yet to fill them with crème. We have the basic outline of the performance therapist and their relationship with the patient. But how can we tell that this is a performance of substance, an authentic performance? Oh, yes, performing authentically – the very core of our piece.

Note

1   See the introduction to Part V.

References

Welling, H. (2018, September 17). Comparing ISTDP and AEDP. 10.31234/osf.io/y2w5c

Greenacre, P. (1954). The role of transference practical considerations in relation to psychoanalytic therapy. *Journal of the American Psychoanalytic Association, 2*(4), 671–684.

Andersen, S.M., & Przybylinski, E. (2012). Experiments on transference in interpersonal relations: Implications for treatment. *Psychotherapy, 49*(3), 370–383. 10.1037/a0029116

Hayman, A. (1990). Some thoughts on the inner world and the environment. Setting the scene. *International Review of Psychoanalysis, 17*, 71–82.

Money-Kyrle, R. (1978) 35. On being a psycho-analyst. *The Collected Papers of Roger Money-Kyrle, 48*, 457–465.

Ingram, D.H. (1993) In these pages .... *American Journal of Psychoanalysis, 53*, 1–2.

Auchincloss, E.L., & Samberg, E. (2012). *Psychoanalytic terms and concepts.* 4th Revised edition. New Haven, Connecticut: Yale University Press.

Lothane, Z. (1995). *Hysteria beyond Freud.* Berkeley: University of California Press.

Lothane, Z. (2009). Dramatology in life, disorder, and psychoanalytic therapy: A further contribution to interpersonal psychoanalysis. *International Forum of Psychoanalysis, 18*(3), 135–148. 10.1080/08037060903116154

Lothane, H.Z. (2011). Dramatology vs. narratology: A new synthesis for psychiatry, psychoanalysis, and interpersonal drama therapy (IDT). *Archives of Psychiatry and Psychotherapy, 13*(4), 29–43.

Freud, S. (1905). Three essays on the theory of sexuality. In J. Strachy & A. Freud (Eds.), *The standard edition of the complete psychological works of Sigmund Freud, Volume VII (1901–1905): A Case of Hysteria, Three Essays on Sexuality and Other Works* (pp. 123–246). London: Hogarth Press.

Green, A. (1975). The analyst, symbolization and absence in the analytic setting (On changes in analytic practice and analytic experience)—In memory of D. W. Winnicott. *International Journal of Psychoanalysis, 56*, 1–22.

Reich, A. (1951). On counter-transference. *International Journal of Psychoanalysis, 32*, 25–31.

Freud, S. (1914). Remembering, repeating and working-through (Further recommendations on the technique of psycho-analysis II). *The standard edition of the complete psychological works of Sigmund Freud, 12*, 145–156.

Reactions [@reactjpg]. (2019). "I pretend I do not see it" [tweet]. Twitter. Web. Retrieved from https://twitter.com/reactjpg/status/1199938361194164224?lang=en

Abram, J., & Hjulmand, K. (1996). The language of Winnicott: A dictionary of Winnicott's use of words. *The Language of Winnicott: A Dictionary of Winnicott's Use of Words, 160*, 1–450.

Bohleber, W., Fonagy, P., Jiménez, J. P., Scarfone, D., Varvin, S., & Zysman, S. (2013). Towards a better use of psychoanalytic concepts: A model illustrated using the concept of enactment. *International Journal of Psychoanalysis, 94*, 501–530.

Pagano C.J. (2012). Exploring the therapist's use of self: Enactments, improvisation and affect in psychodynamic psychotherapy. *American Journal of Psychotherapy, 66*(3), 205–226. 10.1176/appi.psychotherapy.2012.66.3.205

Stern, S. (2016). Enactments in psychoanalysis: Therapeutic benefits. *Psychodynamic Psychiatry, 44*, 281–303.

Boesky, D. (1990). The psychoanalytic process and its components. *Psychoanal Q, 59*, 550–584.

Browning, M.M. (2016). The import of feeling in the organization of mind. *Psychoanalytic Psychology, 33*(2), 284–298.

Winnicott, D.W. (1945). Chapter XII. Primitive emotional development. *Through Paediatrics to Psycho-Analysis, 100*, 145–156.

Karbelnig, A. (2018). Addressing psychoanalysis's post-tower of Babel linguistic challenge: A proposal for a cross-theoretical, clinical nomenclature. *Contemporary Psychoanalysis, 54*, 322–350.

Part IV

Authenticity

We've defined performance art, and we've defined performance art in a psychoanalytic sense. We know how one's identity is performed according to various analytic theorists, and we know how the therapist performs, how they express and execute theory or display and animate their various emotions throughout the session. And we've added the patient to the mix, making our stew ever more flavorful and decadent. But there's one question we haven't necessarily answered. How do we know that the stew is real, made with love and thoughtful care? For all we know, it could be crafted with faux ingredients and simmered for four hours instead of eight. A recipe with seemingly all the right components can taste tolerable and lull us into the misguided belief that we've made something of quality. But how can we be sure that the stew leaves everyone satisfied after the meal is over? To simplify this metaphor: we know performance. But do we know authenticity?

The obvious question here, when speaking of masks worn to the public or idealized senses of self, unattainable or unrecognizable caricatures of one's wishes or fears, is about the therapist's inherent performance automatically constituting inauthenticity. Performativity itself, a factor that may emerge throughout one's practice, is also seen as something inauthentic – a bad word, one that therapists should be avoiding at all costs. Unhealthy features of the False Self, the idealized self, or even unresolved characterizations about the persona can bog down the identity of the performer, making inauthenticity feel very real. And the therapist, performing as a version of themselves that is riddled with conflict, experiences the little unconscious admissions of a repressed identity they don't even know exists.

So it begins! The great discussion on authenticity – and the first problem is defining it. Which of the participants in the therapeutic dyad determines authenticity? Is it the patient, who ideally is the center of most of the dynamic in the relationship? Or is it all chalked up to the transference, or their own core beliefs and conflicts? Is it the therapist, who supposedly knows themselves? If the therapist determines their own authenticity, how can they confront their own lapses in it? Is authenticity simply in the eye of the

DOI: 10.4324/9781003412694-15

beholder – and if it is, who's beholding it? And where did we put those carrots – where are all the carrots?

Now that we're nice and discombobulated, let's revisit the aforementioned topic sentence for some clarity: defining authenticity is inherently a problem. And unfortunately, it's also a necessity. The pursuit of authenticity is important because without it, life at its core remains unfulfilling. Try as one might, if they're consistently crafting a personality that defends against the urges, desires, and feelings they have at their core, this dissonant construction will feel foreign and empty. And the more one tries to force this fabricated facade, the more they'll act out unconsciously as their true wishes bubble up to the surface – whether they want them to or not. Authenticity, much to the contrition of the individual, is not a choice. Inauthenticity, on the other hand, is – though sometimes, it's a choice that your unconscious makes for you after years of consistent behavior, feedback, punishment, or reward.

What we're looking to do here is get a sense of the following: the genesis of authenticity, where it is in the dyad, and finally, how it looks when it's taken out of the frame. Once we see where authenticity comes from and how it forms, we can then bring it out from the individual level and see it exists outside the fortress that is the therapeutic experience. And once we see how a person's truest form is executed and conceptualized in a place of security (meaning the analytic situation), we can see how that authentic self differs, mutates, and conceals itself as it leaves the therapy room behind and enters the world at large. Only then will we know performance – as we'll know what drives it forward.

Where does authenticity come from?

While we now know that authenticity is an internal state of being, we don't know from whence it came. As we've already mentioned, some say that authenticity is borne in childhood, and original desires, fears, and wishes are part of a child's inner fantasy life. As a child grows, these inner fantasies are tamped down by harsh realities, such as misattunements or rejections. And over time, as a means of protecting oneself against the pain of being disappointed, one loses touch with the things they truly wanted early in life. But despite what many might believe about psychoanalysis, finding one's most genuine identity isn't just about regressing to your inner child and unlocking the many things you pined for as an infant. Authenticity evolves as a human does, growing with them as they metamorphize, as they come into being.

There are three things to keep in mind here. Initially, we must remember that how one cultivates an authentic self over their years on earth *isn't a linear journey*. While one can have infantile fantasies that motivate behavior and actions, it's not as if those few beliefs constitute the entirety of your identity. Things occur to you over the course of your life that change who you are, what you believe, and how you behave. Additionally, the various facets of your internal structures, those authentic parts of you that are simultaneously influenced by your past and your present, wax and wane depending on your daily activities.

Just as authentic identity isn't something you climb like a stairway to heavenly self-actualization, it also *isn't static*. Your identity evolves as your life takes shape, and as you move from one stage to another. In childhood, you relate differently to the world than in young adulthood. As a new parent, you see yourself in a different way than you do as an elderly person. And much like your overall identity evolves as you age, your other various identities in life develop at varying paces in varying directions. Much like Erik Erikson's notion of "identity," authenticity is also "never finally 'established' as an 'achievement' but is dynamic and evolves during the course of a person's lifetime both as a function of direct experience of the self and the world and perception of the reactions of others to the self" (Stevens, 1983).

One's identity as a therapist is not precluded from this lifelong journey, and the longer you practice, the more different you'll be from the time you began. A fledgling therapist may go through phases, choosing their identity by cutting some bangs with kitchen scissors and staying out past curfew, or they might wake up one day in their twilight years and realize they've had an identity all along that didn't suit them. Gradually, just as any human being does in life, they'll search for an identity that is authentically theirs. The answers to all of your wants and desires are inside you at all times, but unfortunately for those who prefer stability, these impulses shift and change according to the moment, like items on a seasonal restaurant menu. A sense of authenticity is less about constancy and more about listening to yourself and adjusting accordingly.

As mentioned in the section about identity, the "authentic self" is *not an all-or-nothing experience*. One can have an authentic self, a vulnerable self – your Winnicottian True Self – that needs defenses in order to survive. Without them, the more sensitive authentic bits of you would be too unsafe, resulting in a damaged ego (or worse). And for that matter, the unconscious constantly consists of multiple (and potentially conflictual) thoughts and feelings about any given experience. For every bit of love, there is hate – for every bit of fear, there is excitement – for every bit of isolation, there is longing. All of these feelings are authentic, and though they might be complicated, they all create the whole experience of an identity. So your True Self might not be a hidden thought or feeling, but an intricate amalgamation of many all pureed together into one big soup with flavors and tastes that even you may not be able to put your finger on.

To conclude, the concept of a self is *not just an abstraction*, and authenticity has to weigh one's internal processes with their external environment. Though therapy is helpful in learning more about who one is and why they are that way, there's still the matter of driving the thing you perceive within the frame off the lot and taking it down the highway in the inclement weather of everyday windfalls and pitfalls. The self is a real living thing that you use to interact with the world, whether you're *standing in the space*, as Bromberg put it, of a therapist or a layman. Beres (1981) says that while defining the self as an abstract concept is helpful in therapy, it "cannot be examined in isolation ... it always works with other functions, and evidence of its activity will be found in every action or thought of the person." Everything from the control of instinctual drives to the compromises of id and ego conflicts to symptomologies and pathologies – these are all things that create what Beres calls a "synthetic function" of the self.

This definition of authenticity means the same thing for the therapist as it does for the patient – as it does for any person. In our definition of authenticity in this book (comparable to that of Rousseau's in *Emile)*, we agree that a source from within guides one's true desires, their aims, their wishes, and what will bring them contentedness (1979). It is a supreme good that exists personally, a highly individualized happiness within everyone – an aspiration, a light, a form of sincerity. However, that's about where the comparison ends, as sometimes, that source of authenticity can communicate through the persona, a False Self, or a complicated self-state of the like. A patient's snarky comment in your first year in practice might elicit more countertransference than the same comment would after ten years in the business, or even vice versa. Hearing that a patient suffered a miscarriage might be more striking after you've had children, or helping an elderly patient cope with death might be more painful once you begin grappling with your own mortality. Both of these reactions are truly you. They are who you were, and who you became.

To discern whether or not a therapist's performance is authentic, let us remember that performance is about one's relationship to how they're seen in the world. Our definition is quaint, but it hardly factors in the difficulties of maintaining authenticity in the therapeutic relationship. One could see themselves somewhat realistically, commensurate with how they're seen by others. Or one could see themselves unrealistically, imagining that they're acting in a way they truly aren't – or a little of both could be in the mix depending upon where the therapist is, who they're with, what time of day they're considering or whether they've had their morning coffee. In Bromberg's words, one's ability to sustain "authenticity ... depends on the presence of an ongoing dialectic between separateness and unity of one's self states" (1996). In an ideal situation, when one is running on a full tank of identity, they can recognize the dialogue between varying parts of themselves, able to distinguish "an overarching cognitive and experiential state felt as 'me'," whatever that might feel like (Bromberg, 1996). So though the therapist may be performing, if he has done the hard work to integrate this image into his own ego, there is no value judgment or negotiation on its inherent validity.

That being said, performance can certainly be inauthentic in some cases. Without insight regarding one's internal wishes and desires, one can unfortunately bite into the crunchy crab cake of their behaviors only to find imitation crab meat inside. As Fairbairn says, "the traditional detachment of the analyst (which must be carefully distinguished from the necessary requirement of objectivity of interpretation) has obviously a very high defensive value for the analyst himself" (1958). That is to say, the more the therapist leans on their performance and leans away from their own inner lives, the more likely they are to rest on the laurels of their defenses – defenses that could be preventing them from examining countertransference, which would ultimately benefit the patient.

And what of the patient? Do they notice these nuances, these differences, or the authenticity of the therapist? Are they able to determine authenticity at all, or is the dyad simply too fraught with transference? In these questions we have a bit of an amuse-bouche; we must finish a few more bites of the performance therapist before our next course. However, to tide us over until then, we can make one claim: one need not tell their friends and neighbors that they've eaten enough carrots to turn orange. It shows without any explanation, and without any elaboration. It shows on their skin.

References

Stevens, R. (1983). *Erik Erikson, an introduction/Richard Stevens*. New York: St. Martin's Press.

Beres, D. (1981). Self, identity, and narcissism. *Psychoanalytic Quarterly, 50*, 515–534.

Rousseau J.-J. (1979). *Emile: Or on education*. New York City, NY: Basic Books.

Bromberg, P.M. (1996). Standing in the spaces: The multiplicity of self and the psychoanalytic relationship. *Contemporary Psychoanalysis, 32*(4), 509–535. Web.

Fairbairn, W.D. (1958). On the nature and aims of psycho-analytical treatment. *International Journal of Psychoanalysis, 39*, 374–385.

Chapter 11

Performing a "real relationship"

The performance (nay, the authenticity) of the therapist is not just theoretical, nor is it just emotional – it is practical, and peppered with the varied nuances of the human psyche. The therapeutic frame is designed to be held by the clinician's thoughts, training, and theoretical knowledge. And the therapeutic alliance exists within that frame, one that's messy, unpredictable, and wildly emotional. Though the majority of this manifesto thus far has focused on the performance of the therapist inside of this neat little palatable setting, there's a more complicated component that needs addressing. The therapist and the patient, whether they're inside the therapy room or emailing about a reschedule, have a relationship "notwithstanding the many contrived aspects of the analytic agreement" (Hoffman, 2000). A personal relationship – a non-transference relationship – yes, the real relationship.

The *real relationship* is what some call the interactions that the patient and the therapist have outside of the technical therapeutic relationship. Other therapists call it bunk, or poppycock. To the more well-read psychoanalytic groupies, this concept is not new. The "real relationship" between the patient and the therapist has been long-discussed and long-debated. It fits into what has been named the three-party structure of an analytic relationship (again, with threes!); namely the transference, the working alliance, and the "real relationship" (Greenson, 1967). In short, the working alliance is the relationship, the transference relationship is the relationship within the relationship, and the "real relationship" is the relationship outside of the relationship.

Because the real relationship is free from the restrictions of transference, some equate it with an "authentic" relationship, hence its placement in this section. Rather than putting on the front of a therapeutic persona, a real relationship is seen as a "person-to-person relationship" that differs from a sort of "technical relationship" (Frank, 2005).[1] Unfortunately, Frank continues that the real relationship "is not a concept that has achieved consensual meaning," so much so that the term in literature "is the term in the psychoanalyst's lexicon most regularly appearing in quotation marks" – hence the many quotations marks used above (which were predominantly used to build up to this punch line) (2005). And while believers in the real relationship

DOI: 10.4324/9781003412694-16

(predominantly in the relational field) have attempted to explore the issue, it's still a bit of a mystery. The more traditional analysts believe that it all falls under the transference relationship, which is an inescapable element of the entire therapeutic experience. The real relationship is a slippery slope, they say, and if you begin to classify one interaction as "real," you might be ignoring something that's obviously worth exploring. Others are so convinced as to the real relationship's existence that it's been measured by an inventory; they found that the therapist's negative transference to patients had an impact on their "real relationship" with the patient (Marmorosh et al., 2008). The jury's still out, but the meal must go on. Does this real relationship exist? Does it help? What does it do?

It's "real" complicated

However problematic many of the facets of this concept can be, we're going to operate under the assumption that the real relationship exists – because in many ways, it does, though it's very case-dependent. What it means is slightly altered in every analyst-analysand or therapist-patient dynamic. The old tried and true example of the real relationship is that of the therapist, distanced and observant during the session, who breaks his stance by offering to help an elderly, infirm patient with their coat after the session ends. The clock strikes at 45 minutes, the therapist turns back into a pumpkin (or in this case, a human being), and they're able to interact with their patient in ways that extend beyond the neutrality they're trying so desperately to maintain. The transference relationship ends, and the reality of the patient's infirmity sets in. And the therapist (who in this particular example is a kind person) displays their kindness to the patient by helping in their time of need – unveiling a bit of the man behind the curtain as they do so.

While this definition is reassuringly simple, it's not entirely evocative of the real relationship. The switch that flips a transferential relationship on and off does not operate at the leisure of the therapist, nor at the strike of a clock (Frank, 2005). One could conceptualize that during treatment, the patient constantly sees the therapist as a part object and not a whole one. They only see the therapist in the room, not the entire picture of the individual in all their many self-states. And when the transference is thick, a patient may be so fixed in the phantasy of everything the therapist represents that the idea that they could be a human being in totality is completely inconceivable. Sure, intellectually, the patient is aware that the therapist is indeed a person. But even if these notions don't directly emerge on a conscious level, they're omnipresent on an unconscious level. A therapist getting up to help an infirm patient put on their coat could fill a patient with tenderness and love. It could also fill a patient with unbridled rage or guilt as it shatters some pre-existing image they had of the therapist as their cold, distant caregiver. Or it could mean nothing at all depending on the patient. It's never that easy.

Additionally, distinguishing between what's the real relationship and what is not is extremely muddled – more muddled than helping someone with their coat should ever be. The real relationship isn't designed to be a flaw in the psychoanalytic process; it's a built-in feature. And within the real relationship are certain facts, like a pregnant therapist who must go on maternity leave (Aaron, 1974). The patient isn't having a transference fantasy that the therapist is pregnant; she really is, and that is a real relationship between them. But the feelings that exist parallel to this real relationship are full of content that is specially oriented to the relationship between the therapist and client. To Fairbairn, transference and countertransference exist in the closed system of the analytic space, where the patient's neurosis operates in a predominantly inner reality (1958). And outside of that inner world lies an outer world where the patient must have true relationships with external objects. This is where, ideally, we should conceptualize the real relationship. The fact of the matter is that the therapist is pregnant, and the elderly patient cannot put on the coat on their own. Other facts exist – that a therapist could have maternal characteristics or a kind, good-nature temperament. In the world of the session, these things have deep and profound meanings. And in the world outside the session, they're facts like any others.

Luckily, there's no need to foster a solid real relationship, as it is simply a byproduct of the dynamic (as is the working alliance or the transference). One's real relationship "does not have to be verbalized or conspicuous," though it must be "present to a sufficient degree for the analytic situation to endure the ... often painful process of working through" (Greenson, 1969). One must have faith in the real relationship without pushing too hard for its recognition, as one has faith that the deviled eggs do in fact contain paprika, though sometimes, it resonates in the back of the palate rather than the front. There's also no need for the patient to have the ability to correctly identify attributes of the therapist – how much information they know about the therapist is irrelevant (as we'll speak about when we bring self-disclosure into the mix). What ultimately determines the therapist's engagement with the real relationship, without compromising their therapeutic stance, is their reaction to the patient internally and how that manifests in their words (or sometimes their actions).

In one case written up by sometimes-controversial figure Dr. Ralph Greenson, noted psychiatrist-to-the-stars and father of the modern "real relationship," the line between real relationship and transference is highlighted by a tense moment with an angry patient. The patient compares Greenson to both his wife's analyst and the artist he fantasizes that his wife is flirting with. But he also "indicates some realistic awareness of himself and of [Greenson] as persons," as the patient is well aware that "his reactions are distorted" (1969). In his anger, the patient quite frankly asserts that Greenson "can be wrong, and at times harsh," "warm, not weak," and even "persistent and patient" (1969). These are all things, of Greenson's own admission, fit neatly into a description of himself and his analytic technique. Greenson didn't realize that these facets about himself were being unveiled, but it was seen, internalized, and processed by the patient in a way that led him to truly know the whole Greenson, one that exists in a reality external to the inner world of the dyad. And it led to something productive.

The patient's reactions in the realm of the real relationship were uncovered to "co-exist with transference reactions," and Greenson's addressing of them facilitated "the acceptance of transference interpretations when made" (1969). The patient correctly identifies attributes of his analyst, leading him to a transferential realization about his mother. We see the two things coexist – that the patient is projecting both paternal and maternal feelings on the therapist while also knowing his therapist. Though there is an enmeshment of transference, countertransference, and the "real relationship" that is ultimately co-constructed by Greenson and the patient, the benefit of exploring the patient's insights about Greenson remains the same. In the words of Anna Freud, "analyst and patient are also two real people ... in a real personal relationship to each other. I wonder whether our—at times complete— neglect of this side of the matter is not responsible for some of the hostile reactions [from patients] which we are apt to ascribe to 'true transference' only" (1954).

The performance therapist must keep a sharp eye out for the real relationship, as it can have a profound effect on how treatment goes. Manifestations of the real relationship in meaningful moments can illuminate certain truths about a therapist's performance, and perhaps about the vulnerable self they try to hide behind their therapeutic persona. However, keeping an eye on this complicated feature of the therapy (one of many!) is like juggling the very eggs you'll be deviling – if you focus too much or too little on any one egg, they'll all splat to the ground.

Keeping it "real"

Let's admit it; while it's imperative to remember that real relationships are a part of the performance therapist's repertoire, they aren't easy to examine and navigate. It was Freud who said that the treatment is over when the patient is able to achieve a resolution of their "transference neurosis," meaning that they stop seeing the therapist as an object of pure transference, and start seeing them in a way comparable to the real relationship (Loewald, 1971). But like the succulent flavors of many deliciously intricate curries, the spices and ingredients of each individual therapeutic encounter all blend together to create numerous dishes with many hidden attributes. While one might know the authenticity by taste, it can be hard to pick out how it was made and how it comes about. The process of doing therapy aims to give us a clear view of our dinner party's kitchen, where we can see the chef of our Michelin-starred unconscious add in their various coconut milks and curry pastes. But for the most part, the three-party structure comes out in a dish we've just got to enjoy until we eat it so often that the flavors become known to us. And how the tasty real relationship unveils itself is one of the most subtle flavors of all – almost like one little flavor that pops up time and time again, telling you that there's a dish worth mulling over.

However, many a struggling therapist is interested in getting positive results immediately, mainly good patient outcomes and quick therapist growth. Waiting around for the eventuality that one will understand how their personalities impact their therapeutic performances is rather dolorous, and the pressure to "cure" as quickly as possible comes from all sides.

"The field has been infatuated with and not questioned its emphasis on the rate of recovery," continues social worker Jason Peng (personal communication, 2022). "It's hard to reconcile that since the larger forces at hand – researchers, insurance companies, the field's own experts and luminaries – all seem to tell us to get results as soon as possible."

Consequently, in the attempt to speed up a therapist's insight, the real relationship becomes overpowering. If it's intentionally ignored, it can overwhelm a therapist, who becomes shaken by a patient pointing out aspects of themselves they never recollect unveiling. And if it's overemphasized the therapist begins blurring boundaries with the patient. They then begin priding the real relationship above all else, as they "feel that their uniqueness as a human being is the therapeutic factor in the treatment rather than their knowledge or technique" (Gabbard, 2000). Such examples include Anaïs Nin having sex with her patients on the very couch they used for therapy or Ralph Greenson himself having Marylin Monroe at his home several times a week for champagne and family dinner after therapy (Spoto, 1993). Do as he says, perhaps, but not as he does.

A slippery slope this is, trying to recognize humanity while being mindful about the consequences of overemphasizing it. Sometimes a therapist shows their cards a bit too much, and in a moment, they end up revealing something that causes the patient to see them in a way they didn't want – as a friend, as an enemy, as a nuisance, or as incompetent. The treatment then derails, sometimes for good, and the poor therapist is left to parse out how and why this could have possibly happened; *was it something I said?* But the reasoning is clear: the frenzied practitioner reaches into the cabinet to add a pinch of *self-disclosure*, and in their anxiety, they toss so much in that the dish throws itself away.

Note

1 Which anyone curious about the in-depth history and development of the real relationship should take a look at.

References

Hoffman, I.Z. (2000). At death's door: Therapists and patients as agents. *Psychoanalytic Dialogues, 10*, 823–846.

Greenson, R.R. (1967). *The technique and practice of psychoanalysis*, Volume I (1st ed.). Abingdon, Oxfordshire, UK: Routledge. 10.4324/9780429483417

Frank, K.A. (2005). Toward conceptualizing the personal relationship in therapeutic action: Beyond the "real" relationship. *Psychoanalytic Perspectives, 3*, 15–56.

Marmorosh, C.L., Gelso, C.J., Markin, R.D., Majors, R., Mallery, C., & Choi, J. (2008). The real relationship in psychotherapy: Relationships to adult attachments, working alliance, transference, and therapy outcome. *Journal of Counseling Psychology, 56*, 337–350.

Aaron, R. (1974). The analyst's emotional life during work. *Journal of the American Psychoanalytic Association, 22*, 160–169.

Fairbairn, W.D. (1958). On the nature and aims of psycho-analytical treatment. *International Journal of Psychoanalysis, 39*, 374–385.

Greenson, R.R. (1969). The non-transference relationship in the psychoanalytic situation. *International Journal of Psychoanalysis, 50*, 27–39.

Freud, A. (1954). The widening scope of indications for psychoanalysis—Discussion. *J. Amer. Psychoanal. Assn., 2*, 607–620.

Loewald, H.W. (1971). The transference neurosis: Comments on the concept and the phenomenon. *Journal of the American Psychoanalytic Association, 19*(1), 54–66. 10.1177/000306517101900105.

Gabbard, G.O. (2000). Consultation from the consultant's perspective. *Psychoanalytic Dialogues, 10*, 209–218.

Spoto, D. (1993). *Marilyn Monroe: The biography*. New York: HarperCollins Publishers.

Chapter 12

Self-disclosure and authenticity

Now, where were we? Oh, yes, the dish ran away with itself, and the performance therapist is left pondering the state of things. The structural performance was ideal, the emotional performance was well regulated, and the real relationship was present as a result of those two things being aligned – the therapist felt like an authentic version of themselves in their role. But for just a brief moment, the blinding comforts of the real relationship lulled the therapist into the false assumption that the dyad was a place for *their* perpetual vulnerability just like the patient's. And out came the self-disclosure. Whoops!

Another enlivened discourse fills our dinner party: what is self-disclosure? And what should we think of it? How does the real relationship form if not by human interactions – and how, consequently, is the real relationship folded into the working alliance and transference to create the performance therapist's al fresco? To many, embracing their personhood in the therapeutic frame is a main goal in the performance therapist's process, unequivocally means self-disclosing. Here, we will learn if that really is the case, and if so, what that means for the performing therapist.

What is self-disclosure?

Self-disclosure is defined in many contexts, and it comes in many complex forms. For the most part, the general consensus is that self-disclosures are facts that therapists tell patients about themselves. These facts could be anything from the age of the therapist's child to the reason they canceled a session. Others define self-disclosure as admitting to a patient a feeling, or reaction. This includes telling the patient, "when you were sad, I wanted to put my arm around you and comfort you," or "when you were talking about this topic, I felt myself get sleepy" (Rabin, 2014). And finally, in traditional analytic orthodoxy, even an empathic statement can be thought of as a self-disclosure. Laughing at one of a patient's jokes or crying at one of their stories, to these traditionalists, could be letting down your analytic guard and letting your true self be known – especially if the patient held a predetermined belief that you dispelled with your revelation.

DOI: 10.4324/9781003412694-17

Additionally, self-disclosure is a dirty word to many an therapist. Admitting facts about oneself is seen as breaking the analytic frame, stepping outside, and reorienting the session towards yourself. But in many ways, a self-disclosure is just as much about the moment as the content. We can have self-disclosures that seem innocuous, like what the therapist had for breakfast. Or we can have obviously harmful self-disclosures, such as the [somehow still debated] boundary violation of admitting to sexual feelings about the patient (Davies, 1998). Kohut's previously mentioned handholding could be a self-disclosure – an unspoken confession of caring – and even Freud, who often stressed the need for anonymity, self-disclosed in excess by stressing the importance of his theoretical models directly to the patients he was treating with said models (May, 2008).

Ultimately, self-disclosure, in an all-encompassing, deeply subtle definition, is simply this; informing the patient, consciously, unconsciously, by mistake, or on purpose, of *who you are outside of the confines of their perception of you as a therapist*. It is hinting that the part object is a whole object, implying subtlety that the wizard exists behind the curtain, for better, or even for worse. On an off-day, self-disclosure reveals the therapist as "a good man, but a bad wizard" (Baum, 1939). But are there times when being a good man is better than being a good wizard?

When to self-disclose

The appropriateness of self-disclosure is an enormous conversation. Attempting to delineate what is healthy self-disclosure, where that stands in an analytic frame of neutrality, whether it's helpful or hurtful to a patient, or any of the many other nuances of this topic have long been wrestled over by many a frustrated, bikini-clad therapist in the Jell-O-filled kiddie pool of discourse. And much like many other attributes of analysis, it's rare that two therapists will agree entirely on when self-disclosure is appropriate. Some therapists in the relational or intersubjective schools believe that self-disclosures are absolutely necessary to further the treatment (Ziv-Beiman, 2013). And many modern social worker see self-disclosure as a way they can feel like they're being "transparent" with patients (Knight, 2012). However, self-disclosures of a therapist's psychic state can also morph into harmful enactments where clinicians become aggressive (Walther, 2011) or disengage a patient (Audet & Everall, 2010) – that is to say, inappropriate and boundary-violating.

An inappropriate self-disclosure doesn't necessarily have to be directly harmful or flagrantly bizarre. Alliance-breaking self-disclosures can also seem innocent and harmless, though they may end up lulling the therapist and the patient into a fabricated dynamic of friendship. Take a therapist who shares their gender identity, sex, race, and ethnicity on their Psychology Today profile page in the hopes that a patient with the same demographic information will find them trustworthy, matching the two like a Tinder date orchestrated by the algorithm's kismet. There's definitely something to be said for being culturally competent and connecting with patients from similar perspectives to your own (Soto, 2018). But at present, self-disclosing identities as a way in which to make therapy-skeptical patients more comfortable before the first session even occurs isn't all altruistic, and it presents some larger hidden problems.

"I remember reading American Girl Magazines and seeing that you can get a doll that supposedly looked exactly like you," says social worker Jane Kimmelman in an interview. "If you had blonde hair and green eyes, you could get a doll that had blonde hair and green eyes. But those dolls all had the same face – they don't look like me at all. That's how I feel when people ask for a therapist with the same on-paper identity that they have. It's a facsimile, a set of criteria."

And this "uncanny valley" type of likeness is almost like a defensive structure ready to fail – 'if I find a therapist who's just like me,' the patient thinks, 'they'll understand me without having to explain myself to anyone, including myself.' Furthermore, overidentification with the therapist through these very surface-level characteristics is a ready-made formula for patients to project their own thoughts and feelings about themselves onto the therapist, making transferences and displacements even more difficult to see.

"I don't want to pretend that we don't share the same world," Kimmelman adds. "I'm not an alien, I'm just a therapist." But to likewise pretend that treatment is more likely to succeed because one shares the same skin color or the same gender identity as their patient is just as problematic and generalizing. On the surface it seems so authentic to be vocal about one's demographic information, as it mimics a common understanding of transparency or forthrightness. But disclosing information chosen carefully by a therapist with the express attempt of molding rapport around assumed commonalities is anything but authentic – and it may in fact be performative if a therapist is trying to be culturally competent to prove something to themselves or their peers. And what is a real relationship without authenticity in its self-disclosure? Nothing but a coleslaw with no Dijon mustard – flat and disappointing, leaving one unsatiated, and pining for a little zest.

Ideally, if used at all, the consensus is that good self-disclosure will "contribute to the [therapeutic] process and the patient's therapeutic benefit" and must exist within the context of neutrality (Meissner, 2002). The therapist must be sure that their admissions wouldn't eliminate the opportunity for patients to feel comfortable bringing up any thought or feeling. The aforementioned "inevitable implicit self-disclosure" of "self-revelation" – these natural, humanistic impulses to share – are the centerpiece of the performance therapist's emotional technique (Gediman, 2006). The more unprompted "selective explicit conscious and deliberate self-disclosure" of information about the therapist, Gediman (2006) maintains, is not a part of this equation. The former is the ideal; and the latter is the problem.

Self-disclosure gone awry

First, we'll elucidate on the problem. A good therapist will know when self-disclosure is *patient-centered* with *appropriate boundaries*. Sticking to information that's relevant to the case at hand is key, and maintaining neutrality is paramount. It can be, in fact, dangerous for a patient to hear "unreflective candor" that's ultimately (and very often unconsciously unconsciously) "motivated by countertransference conflicts" (Shill, 2004). Even though the emotions feel genuine, it could also be an unhelpful countertransference enactment, making whatever reassurance the patient feels into yet another convenient and tasty red herring (so many on the menu today!). Whether these admissions are off-the-cuff confessions or individual anecdotes, they need to be pertinent in ways we'll discuss now.

Well-boundaried self-disclosures are in some ways very obvious, but not always. Ralph Greenson having Miss Monroe stay for family dinners is probably one of the most blatant examples of a self-disclosure – disclosing where he lives, disclosing his family's daily goings-on, disclosing that he has a family in the first place! But there are much more nuanced ways that therapists can become unboundaried.

It isn't necessarily just about keeping personal facts to yourself. Some therapists (perhaps in the spirit of the long-dead Fritz Perls or Albert Ellis) have a so-called "tell-it-like-it-is" attitude, where they feel that enabling whatever they consider to be a warped cognition is perhaps a sin of the highest order (Golden, 2021). Instead, they say, they'll blurt out whatever comes to mind no matter how presumptuous it might feel to the patient, citing honesty and authenticity as their driving factors. However, Golden adds that "telling it like it is" can actually be an "anti-intellectual and anti-authority propensity" that enables those who believe they're telling the truth to act out their aggression with percieved impunity (2021). This form of a self-disclosure cracks a more nebulous boundary – an emotional one.

Expressing whatever the therapist might feel in the moment under the guise of honesty (even if it might be invasive or make the patient uncomfortable) is a bit of a simplistic way to look at authenticity. Being authentic doesn't mean being a "truth-teller" or an "open book," as we can recall that this kind of impulsivity within the emotional performance must be leveraged thoughtfully with a structural performance that maintains the value of neutrality. And one who claims that their boundary-breaking forthrightness is for the patient's own good might actually be using self-disclosure as a weapon that crowds out the potential for other perspectives. This is why well-boundaried self-disclosure is so important, and though finding the line between an appropriate and inappropriate one is different with every patient, it mostly comes about through the natural trial-and-error of the therapeutic process.

Patient-centered self-disclosures are the second issue. While it's commonly stated that self-disclosures should be necessary and beneficial, sometimes it can be forgotten for whom the self-disclosure truly benefits. We spoke once of performativity, the notion of exaggerating certain features of oneself in order to maintain an image. Without the therapist getting permission to disclose relevant information, patients feel silenced lose faith in their therapists' professional abilities (Swinden, 2020). Outside the session, one might see a mental health practitioner who posts on social media about serving economically underprivileged populations despite charging $400 a session out-of-pocket. This would be considered performative, as though the therapist may care about the poor, they care slightly more about their paycheck. And in the session, a performative white therapist could be tempted to tell a Black patient all kinds of self-disclosures about their experiences with Black individuals to ensure that the patient is made aware that their therapist is "one of the good ones," so to speak.

Now, we ask ourselves: why would a therapist be driven to these kinds of self-disclosures in the first place? And here we have yet another instance of too many answers – though we'll settle on one here. Think of Horney's idealized image and remember that compulsive unconscious neuroses are ones that are driven by fear rather than out of spontaneity. Rather than listening to a patient's words and responding freely with an empathic response, you might begin to feel your self-disclosures come from a place of anxiety. "I've just *got* to tell this patient my race," you think, "or else they'll feel alienated." "I've just *got* to tell this patient that I'm queer and queer-affirming," you think, "or they'll feel othered by my lack of acknowledgement." Ain (2011) finds that "the relevance of therapist self-disclosure positively correlated with treatment progress" – and if the self-disclosure is therapist-motivated and irrelevant to the patient's needs in the moment, the therapist's mouth is shut and no carrots may enter.

Regretfully, therapist self-disclosures that strive for helpfulness might have the opposite effect, creating a more isolating atmosphere than a welcoming one – even in the contemporary framework of social justice. Unintentionally directing the session by placing importance on these self-disclosures traps you in the same place as the patient: it forecloses on parts of everyone's experience. From the patient's perspective, they feel "silenced" – one interviewee from Swinden's study felt "a lot of loyalty" to a therapist and "didn't really want to challenge him" despite feeling uncomfortable about his self-disclosures (Swinden, 2020). By stepping into a psychodynamic or psychoanalytic therapy room, the environment inherently prides curiosity over judgment. Identities aren't affirmed or denied – rather, they're investigated, studied, and tinkered with. Maybe the patient needs to explore what being queer means to them, and they would feel uncomfortable speaking ill of the community to a queer therapist. If a therapist identifies themselves as a "trans ally" to a transgender patient, the patient is then unconsciously bound to their transness in the dyad, unable to explore a psychic world in which they might enjoy components of their birth gender or have mixed feelings about their transition. Or maybe the patient's anger against other races is a displacement, and by disclosing your own race, you're colluding with them to continue enabling their defense. Ultimately, things that seem important to the therapist may be trivial to the patient, and they could be "very surprised at what in his behavior the patient finds important or unimportant, for the patient's responses will be idiosyncratically determined by the transference" (Gill, 1979). Consequently, disclosures like the ones mentioned above might, in fact, work to serve the therapist (the *idealized* therapist!) who masquerades as someone who's in control of how the patient views them; someone who's able to calm down a patient's anger, relax their anxieties, and reassure their fears, all with just a few demographic facts. But who's anger, anxiety, and fears is this seemingly useful self-disclosure really serving?

To break the fourth wall for a moment: I write a manifesto and I want nothing, yet to say certain things. In an ideal world, the psychodynamic or psychoanalytically minded therapist discloses an identity to the patient in which the patient knows nothing about you, yet they still know who you are. A therapist's race, gender – even pronouns – have no bearing on the treatment unless the patient ascribes them meaning. And even if they do, that meaning continues to be patient-centric, full of transference, and not an arbitrary personal offense to the therapist. The performance therapist does not throw up the carrots he finds nasty or purses his lips like a child refusing dinner. The performance therapist ingests everything and anything they can that will reflect back to the patient. Such is their duty.

This isn't to say that important facets of a patient's personality should be ignored because the therapist is actively omitting explanations of their demographic information from the session. Even if a therapist doesn't plan to self-disclose their race or gender, that doesn't mean that they need to avoid the conversation entirely due to the fear of offending the patient. Would it make a vehemently liberal patient infuriated to be unsure about whether or not their therapist voted for the democratic ticket? Perhaps. But therapy is about exploring the anger by maintaining abstinence, not steering away from the discomfort, rage, and sadness of not knowing by placating the patient's fury. In any other realm, in any other dynamic, this would never occur. But this is the beauty of therapy; that it is a place for these kinds of catharsis, these instances of pure human emotion, joy or mourning, projection and fantasy, to happen.

The perfect coleslaw

Now we come to our recipe: zingy coleslaw with just a touch of Dijon mustard, a way to integrate some of the more complicated parts of the therapeutic experience into a mélange that invokes the real relationship without indulging self-serving self-disclosures. The more delicate and intentional kind of self-disclosure previously mentioned interacts much more fluidly with many different structures of therapy – there are other modalities that embrace self-disclosure no matter what, but we won't be covering those here today. The patient, like a baby looking for reactions from a primary caregiver, is unconsciously and relentlessly assessing the therapist as a means of interpreting their own responses and emotions. Whether these reactions are solely countertransference ones, reflections of the real relationship, or perhaps a combination of the two, the patient internalizes them. And they then feed into the therapeutic alliance.

The performance therapist has a method for this madness. In the psychoanalytic structural performance, the evenly suspended attention should bind one to the patient's thoughts and feelings as they come, the abstinence keeping them from imposing any judgments upon their statements. This "neutrality lies not in the action," Meissner argues, "but in the mental process determining whether the action is appropriate and purposeful" (2002). At the same time, the emotional performance should keep their personhood intact, even as they act in ways that may not come so easy to you in life outside of the therapy room. In terms of unveiling these moments of emotion – self-disclosures, perhaps? – to foster a sort of real relationship bottle-fed by empathy is a foundational part of the performance therapist. And as we've said, to rely too heavily on the structural performance and "to confuse neutrality with anonymity is to deny the inevitability, as well as the psychological necessity, of being oneself" rather than an "artificially contrived, anonymous, professional persona" (Hanly, 1998).

With these components in mind, the therapist can mindfully show themselves to a patient, while also recognizing how that would impact their relationship, and the progress of the therapy. When I laugh with them, does it bring us closer? And why? The patient now knows what you think is funny – and they begin to know you. When something they say surprises me, will it enrage them? And how will we begin to talk about that anger? The patient now knows what you think is surprising – and they begin to know you. And so the arc of every dinner party goes.

Declaiming (oh, there's that word again!) the brave self-disclosure of individual identity beneath one's therapeutic identity is a performance that keeps on giving. But those eggs we're juggling are hard to keep airborne. The issue at hand is to unveil oneself with a counterbalance of technical skill so as to build a relationship that facilitates the growth and insight of the patient. And it's quite simple, really. To do all this, to maintain the whole entire therapeutic performance, one that frames the depth of the real relationship and the shades of the transference relationship with emotion, structure, intimacy, and expertise, the therapist must remember only one thing: be authentic.

References

Rabin, H. (2014). Therapist self-disclosure in individual and group. *Psychotherapy. Group*, *38*(2), 115–125.

Davies, J.M. (1998). Between the disclosure and foreclosure of erotic transfer-encecountertransference: Can psychoanalysis find a place for adult sexuality? *Psychoanalytic Dialogues, 8*, 747–766.

May, U. (2008). Nineteen patients in analysis with Freud (1910–1920). *Am. Imago, 65*(1), 41–105.

Baum, L.F. (1939). *The wonderful wizard of oz.* Oxford, UK: Oxford University Press.

Ziv-Beiman, S. (2013). Therapist self-disclosure as an integrative intervention. *Journal of Psychotherapy Integration, 23*(1), 59–74. 10.1037/a0031783

Knight, C. (2012). Social workers' attitudes towards and engagement in self-disclosure. *Clin. Soc. Work J, 40*, 297–306. 10.1007/s10615-012-0408-z

Soto, A., et al. (2018). Cultural adaptations and therapist multicultural competence: Two meta-analytic reviews. *Journal of Clinical Psychology, 74*(11), 1907–1923. 10.1002/jclp.22679.

Meissner, W.W. (2002). The problem of self-disclosure in psychoanalysis. *Journal of the American Psychoanalytic Association, 50*(3), 827–867.

Gediman, H.K. (2006). Facilitating analysis with implicit and explicit self- disclosures. *Psychoanalytic Dialogues, 16*(3), 241–262.

Shill, M.A. (2004). Analytic neutrality, anonymity, abstinence, and elective self-disclosure. *Journal of the American Psychoanalytic Association, 52*(1), 151–187.

Golden, B. Is 'Tell It like It Is' helpful or harmful? *Psychology Today*, Sussex Publishers, 21 May 2021, https://www.psychologytoday.com/us/blog/overcoming-destructive-anger/202105/is-tell-it-it-is-helpful-or-harmful.

Swinden, C. (2020). The impact of therapist self-disclosure on clients who are them-selves therapists: An exploration of discourse and lived experience. *ChesterRep Home.* University of Chester. https://chesterrep.openrepository.com/handle/10034/623602.

Ain, S.C. (2011). *The real relationship, therapist self-disclosure, and treatment progress: A study of psychotherapy dyads.* College Park, MD, USA: University of Maryland.

Hanly, C. (1998). Reflections on the analyst's self-disclosure. *Psychoanalytic Inquiry, 18*, 550–565.

Audet, C. T., & Everall, R. D. (2010). Therapist self-disclosure and the therapeutic relationship: a phenomenological study from the client perspective. *British Journal of Guidance & Counselling, 38*, 327–34210.1080/03069885.2010.482450.

Gill, M.M. (1979). The analysis of the transference. *Journal of the American Psychoanalytic Association, 27*, 263–288.

Walther, L.D. (2011). When therapists attack: An aggressive instinct in the counter-transference and aggressive behavior in technique. Masters Thesis, Smith College, Northampton, MA. https://scholarworks.smith.edu/theses/1024

Chapter 13

Authenticity and the environment

We've been through authenticity through the perspective of the therapist – the authenticity of their technique through the real relationship and how they express their authenticity in their self-disclosure. But authenticity is not determined by one entire party. It is, ultimately, in the eyes of the co-constructors; that all parties have a say as to whether or not an interaction is candid, as is the case with any other relationship in one's life. Though it is understandable to feel like the patient and the therapist are fundamentally speaking two slightly different metaphysical languages if the patient is nestled firmly in the realm of transference and the therapist is siloed in their bubble of theory, this is a bit short-sighted. Our supposition is that the therapeutic frame is a tripartite one (transference, working alliance, and real relationship) in which both parties exist fluidly. The therapist is always not the arbiter of authenticity just like the patient is not always a rich gravy walled in by the mashed potatoes of their transference. The patient and the therapist are partners in determining "realness ... [which] implies the accurate perception of the other and of oneself", just as their "genuineness ... suggests the ability to be authentic in expression" (McCullough, 2009). And if one party construes the other's reactions as inauthentic, even if they believed themselves to be sincere in their sentiments, the act of genuineness (no matter how formulaic one's structural performance, how restrained their emotional performance, or how real their real relationship) is a moot point. This is why both sides need a say.

As we've said before, authenticity amongst two people can be established in any number of permutations. Authenticity can be a Kohutian holding a patient's hand, or a Freudian abstaining from indulging a patient's provocations. Authenticity can be addressing an awkward moment in the room, or a beautiful moment in the room. But the red thread here, McCullough continues, is that it takes communication to "examine how therapist and patient dyads converge or diverge on the perception of a relationship as real or genuine" (2009). Without the ability to feel the pulse of the room, the shifts and shades, the fluctuation of tenseness and relaxation – and to communicate all of those unspoken auras in a way that's receptive to each individual

DOI: 10.4324/9781003412694-18

patient – the performance therapist cannot perform. This is the way they show their authenticity and create an experience of it: by acting in ways that articulate their most basic curiosities and instincts.

The importance of the therapist's authenticity is that it creates a closed feedback loop, or a kind of "monkey see, monkey do" reaction. Authenticity is mined through subjectivity and synthesized through objectivity – the more the patient gets comfortable with someone who models curiosity, the more they'll be able to explore their transference and internalize external realities that once served as projections. An authentic therapist is one that conscientiously provides a patient with a Winnicottian "holding environment" by signaling to a patient that this is a safe place to know oneself, making a place for connection, communication, sensitivity, and curiosity. Authenticity is about human emotion, human relationships, and human empathy. Authenticity is the art of showing one's personhood. Authenticity is the lifeblood of the performance therapist.

Think of the carrots once again, and how they show on your skin – one cannot mindlessly eat a few as a snack and expect to turn as orange as someone who has been eating dozens of carrots a day for half their lives. To turn orange, one must eat carrots religiously, with intent and assiduousness. To turn orange, one must eat up the transference, the real relationship, the countertransference, the "genuineness," the authenticity – and with purpose and diligence, they will one day show it on their skin in a way only their patients will ever truly know.

Authenticity outside the dyad

While it's all well and good to determine authenticity in the therapeutic frame, as it serves as a tool for the patient to examine their behaviors outside the session, different forms of authenticity manifest throughout different situations in life. Authenticity does not begin and end in the therapeutic encounter, nor is it a definitive state of being. A person's Brombergian self-state changes depending upon how an individual relates to the world and how they *feel* they're relating to the world – their internal barometer for authenticity shifts (1996). And though one's internal life may be vibrant and broad, their external life (or rather, the external environment in which they exist) does alter and change the way they choose to reveal or conceal their vulnerabilities.

The therapist has a peculiar experience of being "authentic" outside of the frame. Seeing patients may in fact help illustrate once-hidden concepts about one's psychic life they didn't know – hence, the entire usefulness of countertransference. But once these revelations are extrapolated from the dyad, they can be hard to grapple with. It especially becomes more difficult when it feels like one's emotional process is the main course of an enormous feast attended by your peers, supervisors, colleagues, and professors.

The therapeutic process isn't just a private and intimate dinner for two anymore, where you and the patient languish over wine pairings and tiny amuse-bouches. This is a buffet, an all-you-can-eat special, and the only way you can become a better chef is to put your most treasured roast recipe out for others to devour and critique. For the therapist, the authentic self must leave the dyad – sometimes sooner than they're prepared for.

Forgoing the metaphor for a moment, the idea is this: whether in a group supervision, a didactic, a social media forum, or a supervision, a therapist's identity is wrapped up in how they communicate and relate to other therapists. There is a prominent wish to seem open and accepting, to come off as well-learned, humble, and ideal. Therapists almost unilaterally agree that their consistent "openness, trust, and devotion" determines if a therapy will succeed (at least those from the sample size of Bitan et al., 2022 do). And oh, these Ideal Therapists who surround you, they have all the passion in the world! They study Bion's algebra equations in their spare time, pursuing continuing medical education credits and debating in book clubs just for the love of the game – how can one keep up? Especially when you recall the enactment you fell into last week, and how your patient canceled their next session. You attempt to turn what you see as a countertransference failure around by embracing it and sharing it in a group as a sort of cautionary tale. But even then, as Boesky says, "it is difficult enough to attempt to describe the complexity of the patient's participation in the psychoanalytic process, let alone to give a truly accurate, honest, and comprehensive account of the subjective experience of the analyst" (1990). Here, authenticity trips and stumbles – admitting publicly one's countertransferential mistakes are "are best, deceptively honest ... superficial and safe, edited versions" or the therapist's thoughts, and "at worst ... exercises in exhibitionistic masochism" (1990). There seems to be no way to win, and you fear that perhaps, you've become – oh, dear heaven – *a bad therapist!*

While these situations might seem familiar, this manifesto is in the business of discussing deeper conceptual meanings rather than distinct scenarios. As such, we must delve into why the therapist's attempt to integrate this very peculiar brand of authenticity into their professional persona is so fraught with emotion. In Freud's world, the social realm is a reflection of our internal conflicts, repressions, and urges for gratification. It becomes "an extension of the ego in its campaign to regulate the drives: cultural leaders are quasi-parents, social forces are camouflaged defenses; group processes are psychodynamics writ large" (Mitchell, 1995). No matter what, one's relationship with society is based in repressing id-driven needs through attempting to have some measure of control over one's environment. This means that authenticity is entirely self-determined, self-motivated, and self-contained. The external world is almost another – let's say it together again! – our third delectable red herring. And if it bothers you, Freud says, you should be looking at your past to find out why.

This traditional view has faced a few contesters throughout the years. The strict infantile drive theory seemed too simple, they argued, and didn't take into account how the external world, including culture and upbringing, can form and shape one's identity. Even Freud admitted that though he wasn't a practicing Jew, this cultural root had an influence "on his 'inner identity' and the independence and clarity of mind which this fostered in the face of majority resistance to his ideas" (Friedman, 1999). Specifically, thoughtful and soft-spoken Erik Erikson did a tremendous amount of work on culture and identity. Identity, Erikson says, is at the "core" of the individual level and the cultural level; an inheritance of sorts that connects the individual with their larger network, "be that section the neighborhood block, an anticipated occupational field, an association of kindred minds, or perhaps (as in the case of G.B. Shaw) the 'mighty dead'" (Erikson, 1968). It is inescapable, unrelenting, a part of every person whose lives it may touch – and even those who denounce it will still be under its "spell" (Stevens, 1983). He calls this process *repudiation*, in which a young person rejects roles or positions that their families or communities deem esteemed; "if a father is a businessman or academic," Stevens continues, "that is the last thing son or daughter will be" (1983).

Erikson's perspective also suggests that because an individual's psychosocial development is based on cultural modes, as a young person develops, their relationship with their identity cultivation, culture, and sense of self can spiral into what he calls an "identity crisis" (1968). Those coming into young adulthood are both battling for and against these cultural puzzle pieces that will invariably shape their lives; they have a "need for freedom yet capacity for discipline, yearning for adventure and love of tradition" (Stevens, 1983). This is where repudiation comes into play. By finding a middle ground between accepting and rejecting one's culture, a sense of self-based in history and context can provide a frame of reference for identity cultivation. And in some ways, like the performance artist needs an audience, the audience of this therapeutic performance are the internalized voices of everyone both the therapist and the patient have encountered throughout life – some that blend together to create soundscapes emphasizing or de-emphasizing certain conflicts that differ within each case.

Identity crises are common, Erikson says, and can be felt in different parts of one's life.[1] Though these identity crises will ultimately "pass with time, empathy, and understanding," Erikson adds that they can be handled by building on the patient's strengths to help them become more self-assured (1968). And if they're not solved (resulting in an *unresolved identity crisis*), an unsure teen can become a lost adult. They become someone constantly seeking an identity that's opposed to or in line with their worldview. But that worldview feels rejecting and isolating either way, and the individual feels socially and psychically inaccessible.

As for how this relates to authenticity, performance, and the therapist's life outside the dyad, follow along here. It's said that Erikson and our old friend

Winnicott had "remarkable theoretical similarities;" Winnicott himself "recalled very generally how Erikson's propensity to work with a patient's strengths had strongly influenced his own clinical work" (Friedman, 1999). And here, we can see someone who becomes an actor by building out a visage to safeguard an unformed self, unsure of its own desires. While the inner self is free to have identity crises that remain unresolved, the outer self, the one that relates to the world, can be whatever its culture expects of it without having to look inward at the complicated feelings that might stir up. The performance of the compliant False Self, the confused authentic yearnings of the confused True Self – the therapist is suddenly not just in an Oedipal struggle with their supervisor. Informed by their specific upbringing, they're trying to decide whether they want to be him or be the opposite of him.

The solution to the authenticity problem?

So the therapist explores their own authenticity on a personal level, attempts to make sense of it in the dyad as they balance their structural performance with their emotional one, and *also* must grapple with idea that the whole *world* of therapy is a macrocosm of all the various situations one might encounter in their own practice. In some ways, it's hard to imagine how a therapist wouldn't have an identity crisis at one point or another in the attempt to keep this busy kitchen functioning without a hitch. How overwhelming, to be trapped in a cycle of discovering the authenticity beneath one's performance – or the authentic parts of your performance – just to feel that they're subject to study, review, and dissection time and time again in a formal work-centered context as well as a personal one. Discovering and working through authenticity comes with baggage, some of which is so brittle that you have an urge to keep it concealed from others. Certain wishes and desires might conflict with the False Self, persona, or idealized image that one constructs to acclimate to certain situations they frequently find themselves in. When broken down this much, it seems like quite the conundrum. How can a profession this difficult be made easy?

We've been through this before. Authenticity is connection, communication, sensitivity, curiosity; human emotion, human relationships, and human empathy. Freud's understanding of a realized patient is one who has autonomy and freedom despite reality-based constraints. In his own words, the goal of treatment wasn't to completely cure a patient of all symptoms, but to "give the patient's ego freedom to decide one way or the other" (1923). This performance therapist of which we speak is not one who lends moral value judgments to a patient's feelings; this performance therapist "respects a patient's individuality and does not seek to remold him in accordance with his own personal ideals" (1923). The patient then isn't shackled by their imposing superegos or impulsive ids, and their ego feels free to act in a way that balances self-control and self-expression. And much like Winnicott's infant, who needs a relative amount of subjective omnipotence to establish a sense of control over their realities, this ability to feel even a modicum of sovereignty over their own psychic realms can prevent a hopeless or helpful mindset from developing later in life. And what is connection, sensitivity, and curiosity but a choice to push forward through defenses and into another's personhood? If the patient's "power of initiative" is one of the most important dimensions of one's sense of self, why isn't the therapist's (Freud, 1923)?

The therapy room is a place for exploration – for one's therapeutic identity to develop as much as the patient's does. The performance therapist sees therapy like he sees this manifesto – a jaunt, an investigation, a place to survey and muse about the choices they make in their practice. Only when this performance therapist allows themselves to frolic in the fantasy space will they see everything align. The structural performance taught them the recipe. The emotional performance grew the ingredients. The real relationship brought the patient's ingredients along. And the environment closed the loop as the performance therapist brings out their beloved dish, fit for a feast of other expertly trained performance therapists, with tips and tricks that will feed back into their structure. The process goes on as long as one practices – they continue to wonder, discover, evaluate, and evolve. Their identities congeal and mature until patients come from far and wide to make exciting new meals with this famed connoisseur. And we move back into the garden of conjecture for our dessert – as our reward for all our hard work, we've finally come into being.

Note

1   To learn more about that, look into Erikson's Eight Stages of Psychosocial Development (Bishop & Keth, 2013; Bishop, 2013).

References

McCullough, L. (2009). The challenge of distinguishing figure from ground: Reaction to Gelso's work on the real relationship. *Psychotherapy Research, 19*, 265–268.

Bromberg, P.M. (1996). Standing in the spaces: The multiplicity of self and the psychoanalytic relationship. *Contemporary Psychoanalysis, 32*(4), 509–535. Web.

Bitan, T., et al. (2022). Therapists' views of mechanisms of change in psychotherapy: A mixed-method approach. *Frontiers in Psychology, 13*, 10.3389/fpsyg.2022.565800.

Boesky, D. (1990). The psychoanalytic process and its components. *Psychoanal Q, 59*, 550–584.

Mitchell, S.A., & Black, M.J. (1995). *Freud and beyond: A history of modern psychoanalytic thought*. New York City, NY: Basic Books.

Friedman, L. (1999). *Identity's architect: A biography of Erik H. Erikson / Lawrence J. Friedman*. New York: Scribner.

Erikson, E.H. (1968). *Identity: Youth and crisis*. New York City: Norton.

Stevens, R. (1983). *Erik Erikson, an introduction / Richard Stevens.* New York: St. Martin's Press.

Bishop, C., & Keth, K. (2013). Psychosocial stages of development. 10.1002/978111 8339893.wbeccp441.

Freud, S. (1923). The ego and the id (1923). *TACD Journal, 17*(1), 5–22, 10.1080/ 1046171X.1989.12034344

Bishop, C.L. (2013). Psychosocial Stages of Development. The Encyclopedia of Cross-Cultural Psychology, 1055–1061

Part V

Application

And as we've gotten in the habit of doing, we've opened another can of worms; these, however, are the tastiest and most important part of our meal – what both Zagat and the New Yorker recommended we try while we're here. We've done a great job of reading up on how the performance therapist looks, what constitutes a performance therapist, and how authenticity informs his practice. But now the performance therapist is served on fine china for our salivating palates, and we still have so many more questions. Who on earth is the performance therapist – one who accepts the doctrine of integrating performance and authenticity? Can he finally and definitively answer this question for his patients – the question of the performative and the authentic? As we've said before, they're oxymoronic on the surface, and seem hardly to work in tandem. A performance: a supposed display of acting as a character – a non-self, an "other," a cover, a shield. A funhouse mirror that relays facets of the authentic self in contortions and distortions, turning one's external presentation into an exaggeration. The authentic: the vulnerable reality of someone's inner life, or the truth of who they really are. A performance is the protection of the authentic. A performance relays the authentic without un-veiling too much. In many ways, a performance *is* authentic if it's done with intentionality. We know this already. But a new question now graces our palates: *what do we do with the performance therapist now that we've made him?*

Dessert is served

The performance therapist, should he choose to accept this manifesto as his own, has a goal – much like that of the performance artist. If we can recall from all those pages ago, the performance artist is one who seeks to physically embody a notion they feel empowered to disperse, whether it's political, personal, or for the sake of questioning the totality of art as a concept. And like them, the true performance therapist feels compelled, in the way that the artist is, to relay to their patients the nuances and existential elements of therapy – something they've spent so long cultivating. In this, the therapist goes from just a person bearing witness to their fellow man to an *idea*, a

DOI: 10.4324/9781003412694-19

specific philosophy incarnate, informed by their own thoughts, feelings, and study, guiding another through the peaks and valleys of their own psyche. That is their goal. To do, and to be.

The manifesto of the performance therapist is now clear. We've identified the components of this creature, explored their meaning, and shown their process. But now, we must examine how they manifest, and who, in fact, qualifies for membership into this seemingly elite club. Seemingly, we say, because despite all the naval-contemplating over what is and what isn't, the performance therapist is not an intentional identity. Rather, it is an inherent one. It is claimed simply by being a therapist, or therapist-in-training, or any of the other mental health practitioners mentioned earlier in this piece. They are someone who agrees that they seek all the things a performance therapist seeks, believing all that they believe – that a structural performance and an emotional performance are best learned, practiced, and executed when leveraged with an authentic relationship fueled by one's knowledge of oneself. They need not have the presence of mind to *call* themselves a performance therapist, but they certainly can. They can also reject the label, if they see fit, if the performance therapist mentality doesn't fit within the foundations of their practice. And there may be variations – the performance social worker, the performance clinical psychologist, the performance mental health counselor (a mouthful!) – perhaps also bound together by various common structural frames.

We know another performer who treats their label the same way. Just like in performance art, there are truly no prerequisites to be a performance artist; the category of "artist" is still applied, despite the technique used or intention behind the work. To be a performance artist, one can either thoughtfully craft the duct-taped banana to the wall of Art Basel, requiring an eye for aesthetics; or one can eat it, with only a hand to hold, a hand to peel, an empty stomach, and a commentary in mind. Rejecting the label or embracing it does nothing for the performance artist – as Howell says, these two fields are tied together by action of "positing an enquiry into [performance's] own essential nature" (2000). And so, the performance therapist and the performance artist may choose to exist together quietly, without all the hullabaloo and fanfare other performers sometimes enjoy.

Here we'll have another refresher, as I'm sure we're forgotten all about the art and science debate of so many chapters ago. How the performance therapist defines themselves comes solely from both how they see their own therapeutic practices and therapy on the whole – not from the definition of a performance therapist itself. We can have a performance therapist who thinks of himself as a scientist, removed and distant, with only inquiry driving him, or we can have a performance therapist who is already an artist, a painter, a poet in his other life; one who brings with him the identity of artist to all work he does. It can be a deeply personal experience, guarded in secret, or one discussed among peers and supervisors in an attempt to sort through the notion of identity with lively discourse. As long as one is an actively practicing therapist, this identity is theirs.

The secret sauce of the "good enough" performance therapist

And so our little model, our little homunculus, has made his big debut. We can be him or not be him, love him or hate him, spit him out, or swallow him whole. But as we stare at our creation, the guest of honor at our lovely dinner party, a voice pipes up from the end of the table. This is, of course, the moment where any reasonably minded person in the field of therapy slaps their hand to their head in exasperated anguish (if they haven't done so already, as there have truly been some tasteless comments throughout this work). 'Of course, you numbskull!' you say to yourself, pointing wildly at the performance therapist. 'This is why I went to years of personal therapy and training – the core of the performance therapist is the aspiration of integrating theory into practice.' But, of course, it's never that simple. Going, reading, and learning is only half the battle, and for the performance therapist, the end goal isn't necessarily to be a perfectly integrated mental health practitioner (primarily because it's an unachievable goal). It's entirely possible to be able to pass a test not only on theory, but on your own ego defenses, drives, and object-relationships – and in the same metaphorical breath, be so consumed by your own pathology that you lose track of the inevitable elements of attachment and humanism in this work.[1] The goal of the performance therapist is not just to do, but to be; not to achieve, but to exist.

There is a secret sauce in the performance artist made only with the complicated ingredient of time, comparable to the patience required in allowing the real relationship to blossom. The performance therapist must wear this label throughout life, never forgoing their mission: bettering their performance through professional and personal exploration. Expertise cultivated through a particular set of channels, such as supervision, education, and mindful practice, rather than just hours of experience, is substantiated by data (Hill et al., 2017). The régime of the performance therapist requires a perfect marination time and blend of spices to coat the beef ribs of the therapeutic process. But every case is different, and though you may hone your recipe over time, you can always tweak it depending on whichever ingredients the patient brings. This is not a performance that lasts 90 minutes with one intermission. This is a performance that lasts a lifetime.

Even if some level of expertise is the goal for the performance therapist, they should not lose sight of the performances they complete on a day-to-day basis. Like Winnicott's "good-enough mother," the "good-enough performance therapists" are out there (1986). The ideal performance therapists are what the literature calls "master therapists" – "voracious learners," those who "use both experience and intelligence" to be "quite reflective and self-aware," possessing "emotional maturity and strength of character that come from years of active learning and living" (Jennings & Skovholt, 1999). One who can constantly and perfectly balance empathy and intuition with training and intellect. But is it always the reality? What of those who wish to walk the road of ultimate understanding, of literature and connection, empathy and intelligence, but don't know how, or are hindered by their own conflicts? Those with no money to endure long and strenuous analytic training, those with a poor psychodynamic education, or those inclined to self-disclosures or loose boundaries? Those who get wrapped up in enactments, in acting out, in sticky countertransferential situations? "It is wise to be aware of how easily we can become de-skilled," says Cooper (1986). "Our emotional investment in each of our patients is large, our propensity for disappointment is great, and our opportunities for reward are deliberately limited. operate in a climate of extraordinary isolation." Does the weight of their imperfections render them helpless – and render their patients unhelped?

Those working towards the ideal also suffer the unfortunate fate of living in the unknown, clawing desperately at attempts to understand the psyche, and the conditions of existing. working through of the performance therapist requires a delicate combination of their own therapy, their practice, their supervision, and their study. But "the desire to be a good analyst makes it difficult to be an analyst" (Micati, 2008). This is why we have the performance therapists. After all is said and done, after thousands of words and thousands of thoughts, we look at the end of the table and see a sweet little man having a lovely dinner. The performance therapist isn't wringing his hands, wondering if he'll be good enough. He is merely performing his personhood for all party attendees to enjoy. A much simpler identity than it seems, a performance therapist just is. Inquisitive, empathic, authentic. That's all there is to it.

Viola! Magnifique!

We'll soon wrap up, but don't worry – everyone gets a recipe booklet of their own to take home, so that you may try some of these dishes out for yourself. However, you should anticipate that the process will taste dramatically different in real life than it did during the party. In its execution, the performance of therapy creates nuance in the dyad beyond just their organic interplay. This new combination of performing artist and therapist has an almost endless potential for experimentation, assessment, and even academic probing. The intersectional possibilities are endless – though we only have so many pages here.

The embalming of psychotherapy and performance art into one cohesive field of study illuminates particular notions, like colors in the refracted light of a Baked Alaska. Performance is red, analysis is yellow, and the blend creates orange; a spectrum of many oranges, in fact, that all fashion a beautiful array of colors to explore. It seems apt, here, to finish off such a manifesto by staring into the flames and making meaning of them. This identity was borne from the nearly absurd, incorporeal perspectives of anti-establishment, anti-art, anti-everything. Invented out of an incapability of other modalities of patient care to provide comfort and symptom relief. Different in every performance, unrepresentable by words or by pictures. What is at stake here by looking at the character of the therapist – at the entire process of therapy – as something so imprecise? What did we make, what did we do? How does it endure? How does it exist in this unnamable, chaotic, impassioned, and unspeakable form? And in the big picture of the therapeutic performance, how do we begin to define this metaphysical contribution more inexplicably philosophical than any other relationship? The mystery of the human connection, the magic of relating – perhaps, the coming into being?

Note

1   I know this to be true from an off-the-record interview – but understandably, the psychiatrist who admitted such a thing wished to remain anonymous.

References

Howell, A. (2000). *The analysis of performance art: A guide to its theory and practice* (1st ed.). Abingdon, Oxfordshire, UK: Routledge. 10.4324/9781315079813

Hill, C.E., Spiegel, S.B., Hoffman, M.A., Kivlighan, D.M., & Gelso, C.J. (2017). Therapist expertise in psychotherapy revisited. *The Counseling Psychologist*, *45*(1), 7–53. 10.1177/0011000016641192

Winnicott, D.W. (1986). The theory of the parent-infant relationship. In Buckley, P. (Ed.), *Essential papers on object relations* (pp. 233–253). Location, New York City, NY: New York University Press.

Jennings, L., & Skovholt, T.M. (1999). The cognitive, emotional, and relational characteristics of master therapists. *Journal of Counseling Psychology*, *46*(1), 3.

Cooper, A.M. (1986). Some limitations on therapeutic effectiveness: The "Burnout Syndrome" in psychoanalysts. *Psychoanalytic Quarterly*, *55*, 576–598.

Micati, L. (2008). The experience of supervision. *The Italian Psychoanalytic Annual*, *2*, 73–87.

Chapter 14

Coming into being
(or, the magic of relating)

It took us quite a while, but we've gotten to the subtitle: coming into being (as, of course, the title itself must be much less metaphorical and much more oriented toward keywords). The final product of mixing performance art and therapy (in this context, performance art and psychoanalysis) – the odd mix of thoughts and feelings someone experiences when they walk into a gallery and see a man rip a duct-taped banana off of the wall to eat it. It is the watching and experiencing of performance art, the act of discovering and processing it from within, feeling it all come together in the particular place and time it occurs. It is beyond description; sometimes, beyond comprehension. But creating the magic of relating is an active process; "when anything comes into being which did not exist before," Diotima says in Plato's Symposium, "the cause of this is always composition" (2001). It is a fundamental product of the performance therapist's work; it is the thing that elevates their work from casual to intentional. It is completely incontestable and almost incomprehensible. One could call it the beauty of intimacy, the mystery of being known and knowing, immersion in the tableau, a cathexis to the whole therapeutic process – any of the above or none at all. In a nonsensical, Dadaist way, the patient and therapist play around in the psychic space, and as the therapist tries to internalize, process, and reflect this play, the two make meaning from the human experience, however illogical it might seem.

Something like this experience has been dubbed "the Third" by relational theorists such as Lew Aron (2006), comparable almost to an observing ego, a place in which the system develops agency, and becomes a subject in the therapy (Mills, 2017). While not a strictly relational sentiment, as this unfathomable bond is not the entire groundwork of the therapeutic relationship, the natural organism of the therapeutic process becoming an unspoken presence in the room and is prevalent in any therapy, psychoanalytic or otherwise. And that organism comes to life with the cherished connection that feeds it – a connection built upon a performance therapist who invests in their performance.

The label of "coming into being" is certainly not a novel concept – in fact, it's a phrase Thomas Ogden says relatively regularly. Ogden's general

DOI: 10.4324/9781003412694-20

definition was more about the patient's independent development in the holding environment as they begin to wean themselves from whichever figure – mother, therapist, caregiver – is providing that environment for them (Ogden, 1986; Bram & Gabbard, 2001). However, he also uses it more colloquially as a way to refer to one's personal evolution. The therapeutic (namely, the analytic) process is essentially invented over and over with every patient, he says; in transforming the works of past theorists into "our own, we are coming into being as thinkers in our own right, whose ideas others in the future will make use of in the process of creating themselves in ways that are unimaginable to us now" (Ogden & Donna, 2013; Ogden, 2021).

Here, our definition of coming into being and the magic of relating is a bit different. If everything aligns for the performance therapist, the magic of relating is the venue he will perform in; the Volkswagen he will crucify himself on, the tree he will climb naked, the room he will sit in for hours on end as others come and sit with him (Burden, 1974; Schneemann, 1976; Abramović, 2010). We take the performance therapist off the page and put him into the room with the patient – and coming into being is what we see. This strange scene is not directly about aesthetics, nor is it solely about the emotional work. It rather is the amalgamation of emotions, relationships, transference and countertransference, mood, room, wallpaper and hairstyles, outfits and furniture, temperature, taste and smell, all into something inexplicable. To Agger, the session was "reciprocally affected by" small things, such as "physiological responses, behavioral anomalies, and sensory images that are evoked or spontaneously generated either within the analytic setting or outside during the course of my presumedly personal life" (1993). And this is the performance. The authentic performance.

We call it coming into being (or, the magic of relating) because we do not know what else to call it. This is not to say this phenomenon can never have a name, or that there aren't very specific components and details that create the finished product (in fact, we've been over many thus far). And furthermore, this world is not an unknown one to the skilled therapist, whether or not they're practicing as a performance therapist without the label to tout. They know the unspoken sense of reality, this dream-like co-construction, this feeling that binds them to the work in the day-to-day. Marina Abramović said herself, regarding The Artist is Present, "nobody could imagine … that anybody would take time to sit and just engage in mutual gaze with me" in total silence, and to see those across from her crying, laughing, and sharing a strange form of intimacy "was [a] complete surprise" (Zec, 2013). In therapy, this is the norm; to sit and be with someone, to bear witness to them. The therapy is the performance art, their many patients revolve in and out of the extra chair as the collective unconscious audience watches from the roped-off halls of the MoMA. More often than not, the therapeutic dyad "provides a terrain for expressing the language of the emotionality experienced by the analytic pair in an intimate relationship" (Levy, 2017). This uneasy potential,

Levy argues, for riding the waves of emotions alongside patients, "is what allows us to access the patient's intimacy and our intimacy ... facilitating the emergence of an experience of truth and beauty, outside exclusively rational parameters" (2017). Within the walls of the session, the therapist and patient are almost free to craft their own reality, one of fantasy and closeness, familiarity and peculiarity. A bond that's as difficult to put into words as the language of a Hugo Ball poem.

Call to mind, again, the image of The Ideal Therapist: is he looking at you with scorn, or with pride, when he sees how you acknowledge this delicate union, to your peers, in your writing, to your patient themselves? Does The Ideal Therapist see two scientists on a journey of hypotheses and investigation? Does he see the incredible, unnamable, and ethereal presence in the bond you are sharing with the patient, and sharing with the world? And, more importantly, separate from this persona ripe with your own personal conflict, the persona that casts a fog over your own therapeutic identity, what do *you* see?

The therapist performs with the eyes of their patients and the field upon them – they perform in tweed jackets, in cardigans, in midcentury-modern offices, in old, dusty institutions, and shiny new group practices. All of these therapeutic relationships are deep, meaningful interactions held with other human beings, uniting them through more than just surface-value tokens of bonding. In some ways, just as therapists know and understand their patients, the patients will eventually come to know and understand a therapist on a more attuned level than either of them realize. These therapists – these performance therapists – are all therapists before them, and all therapists after them. They are all the practitioners they wish they could be and all the practitioners they fear they could be. Some of a more Jungian perspective may know it as the collective unconscious. Today, we call it a part of our dessert.

Many already recognize that the therapeutic alliance is thoroughly intimate or expressive, and it may be difficult to sit back, embrace the performance, and take a metaphorical lighthearted stroll through something so powerful. Therapy can often be a solemn, intense, and high-stakes experience. But as the party clears and we mosey around the garden of conjecture, enjoying the stunning surroundings and wonderful aftermath of good wine, good food, and good company, we must also enjoy it. The therapeutic performance can be fun, light, and humorous – it can be aggressive, awkward, and irritating. It can be the spectrum of human emotions, and ideally, it *will* be. By learning to embrace the authentic performance as something beyond the grave seriousness of their work, a therapist can enjoy this thing worth enjoying: coming into being, the magic of relating. And in all the joy, agony, sadness and hilarity of the human condition, performing becomes easy.

This "internal negotiation with the realities, values, affects, and perspectives," again in the words of Bromberg, allows for cohesion; rarely should one specific facet of the self "function totally ... without the participation of the other parts of self" (1996). The performance therapist gets up from the dinner table and does this little self-state shuffle; one step towards recognizing their performance, one step into assuming and integrating that role, and one little shuffle-ball-change into the realm of silly realism. A therapist who sees themselves for who they really are will find themselves liberated from the somber shackles of their own making – shackles that tie them to an Ideal Therapist they do not want to be. This was the essence of Dadaism, of Futurism, and the beginnings of performance art: to embrace this absurdist notion of life through one's own commentary on it.

The irony of this whole work is not lost on the fact that spelunking into the human experience is inherently limited in ways parallel to its own criticisms. The contemporary performance artwork *Iris: A Space Opera* cites this very sentiment in a way; to record a concert distinctly removes the tableau crafted by an audience's interaction with an artist, and to watch it on a screen almost does a disservice to the experience (Chemetoff & Beraud, 2019). In this manifesto, we are recording a concert, capturing the sweat, throbbing ear drums and sore feet, adrenaline and revelation, as we sit in the movie theater, nestled in our air-conditioned simulation with a warm bag of popcorn. The attempted emulation of an experience without one's presence within it cannot compare to the reality. And likewise, no matter how much we read of the performance therapist, the absolutely ethereal enchantment of the therapeutic experience is never known until you're there, in the room, living through it with someone else.

It's been quite a lovely dinner, and I hope you're satisfied. The performance therapist waves goodnight and leaves with one final parting gift: a declamation. We know now how to attempt the unveiling of one's thoughts, feelings, and philosophies about the mind without ever unveiling ourselves – like Tzara, we have successfully created an "abolition of logic" (1918). We know how to give a patient everything, and nothing at all. To show them who you are without ever telling them anything – to silently feast on the carrots they offer you, and to show it on your very *skin*. To speak to them in a language of words you both created, to sit with them in peace and solace – to defy the rules of conventional thought, feeling, and relationships. To perform to the highest standard of their degree. To perform – to purely and authentically perform. For them, and for yourselves.

References

Plato, Benardete S., & Bloom A. (2001). *Plato's symposium*. Chicago, IL, USA: University of Chicago Press.

Aron, L. (2006). Analytic impasse and the third: Clinical implications of intersubjectivity theory. *International Journal of Psycho-Analysis, 87*, 349–368.

Mills, J. (2017). Challenging relational psychoanalysis: A critique of postmodernism and analyst self-disclosure. *Psychoanalytic Perspectives*, *14*(3), 313–335.

Ogden, T.H. (1986). *The matrix of the mind: Object relations and the psychoanalytic dialogue*. Northvale, NJ: Aronson.

Bram, A.D., & Gabbard, G.O. (2001). Potential space and reflective functioning: Towards conceptual clarification and preliminary clinical implications. *International Journal of Psychoanalysis*, *82*, 685–699.

Ogden, T.H. (2021). *Coming to life in the consulting room: Toward a new analytic sensibility* (1st ed.). Abingdon, Oxfordshire, UK: Routledge. 10.4324/978100322 8462

Ogden, T.H., & Donna, L.D. (2013). Thomas H. Ogden in conversation with Luca Di Donna. *Rivista di Psicoanalisi*, *59*, 625–641.

Burden, C. (1974). *Trans-Fixed [Performance]*. Venice, California.

Schneemann, C. (1976). *Up to and including her limits*. Madrid: Museo Nacional Centro Reina Sofia. Web.

Abramović. (2010). *The artist is present*. New York: MoMA. Web.

Agger, E.M. (1993) The analyst's ego. *Psychoanalytic Inquiry*, *13*, 403–424.

Zec, M. (Director). (2013). *Marina abramović: Early years*. [Video] Hudson, NY: Marina Abramovicć Institute. Web.

Levy, R. (2017). Intimacy: The drama and beauty of encountering the other. *The International Journal of Psychoanalysis*, *98*(3), 877–894. 10.1111/17458315.12681

Bromberg, P.M. (1996). Standing in the spaces: The multiplicity of self and the psychoanalytic relationship. *Contemporary Psychoanalysis*, *32*(4), 509–535. Web.

Chemetoff, A., & Beraud, A. (Directors). de Gunzbourg, H., & Tenneroni, M. (Producers). (2019). *IRIS: A space opera by justice*. [Video/DVD] Paris, France: Pathé. Web.

Tzara. (1918). *Dada manifesto*. Zurich, Switzerland: Cabaret Voltaire. Web.

Index

For Product Safety Concerns and Information please contact our EU
representative GPSR@taylorandfrancis.com
Taylor & Francis Verlag GmbH, Kaufingerstraße 24, 80331 München, Germany

www.ingramcontent.com/pod-product-compliance
Lightning Source LLC
Chambersburg PA
CBHW052013270326
41929CB00015B/2898